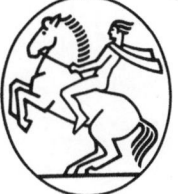

H. Resch and E. Beck (eds.)

Arthroscopy of the Shoulder

Diagnosis and Therapy

Translated from the German by M.-L. Antoft
and B. Marschall

Springer-Verlag Wien New York

Dr. Herbert Resch
Dr. Emil Beck
Universitätsklinik für Unfallchirurgie
Innsbruck, Austria

With 125 Figures (63 in color)

ISBN-13:978-3-7091-9205-4   e-ISBN-13:978-3-7091-9203-0
DOI: 10.1007/978-3-7091-9203-0

Preface

In the last few years arthroscopy has been firmly established as an investigative and therapeutic modality with regard to the knee and more recently to the shoulder joint. The establishment of a clinical diagnosis in the shoulder joint can be a difficult problem, as the site of the symptoms only very rarely coincides with the area of the actual lesion. Diagnostic arthroscopy together with other imaging techniques has greatly contributed to the assignment of symptoms to particular lesions. Direct visualization of the intraarticular structures provides clear and precise information in both normal and pathological conditions. Visual exploration on the intraarticular structures allows arthroscopy to be used as a means of diagnosis also in the soft tissue layer of the soulder joint. The thick soft tissue layer surrounding the shoulder joint, in particular, presents a challenge to avoid open surgery, as arthroscopic surgery shortens the postoperative rehabilitation time. This is why a variety of therapeutic techniques in the field of arthroscopic surgery have been and are still being intensively researched. Several methods have already become routine. Bankart refixation techniques as well as techniques for arthroscopic acromioplasty are two examples.

This brings us to mention the excellent cooperation provided by members of the Institute of Anatomy of the University of Innsbruck. We would also like to thank the head of the institute, Prof. Dr. W. Platzer, for his generous support in founding an arthroscopic laboratory for research in his department. Some of the already existing arthroscopic surgical techniques were improved and new ones developed in this laboratory.

The primary objective of this book is to provide comprehensive information on the latest developments in diagnostic and therapeutic arthroscopy. We have tried to include as much practical information as possible, much of it gained from trial and error experience in our department, but also gleaned from published reports and personal communications with other surgeons.

A wide range of illustrations hopefully assists comprehension of the text and, in particular, illustrates the individual operative steps. Furthermore, we considered it important to emphasize the indications for arthroscopic surgery and the preoperative assessment has been given considerable attention.

The manuscript was translated by Marie-Louise Antoft and Brigitte Marschall. The editors gratefully acknowledge the assistance by Dr. Roger Butorac, F.R.A.C.S., Salt Lake City, Utah in the editing of this volume and express their appreciation to Dr. Robert A. Balyk, F.R.C.S., Edmonton, Alberta and Dr. Tim Briggs, London for reviewing the translation.

Innsbruck, May 1992   H. Resch and E. Beck

Contents

List of contributors

M. Lener
H. Maurer
Institut für Anatomie der Universität Innsbruck, Innsbruck, Austria

I. Braito
R. Habeler
Universitätsklinik für Anästhesie und Intensivmedizin, Innsbruck, Austria

W. Glötzer
K. Golser
A. Kathrein
H. Resch
G. Sperner
H. Thöni
Universitätsklinik für Unfallchirurgie, Innsbruck, Austria

P. Habermeyer
E. Wiedemann
Klinikum Innenstadt, Ludwig-Maximilians-Universität, Munich,
Federal Republic of Germany

R. Butorac
Division of Orthopedics, University of Utah Medical Center, Salt Lake City, Utah, USA

Drawings by C. Konzett, Dornbirn, Austria und S. Mills, Munich,
Federal Republic of Germany

1 Anatomy of the shoulder joint

H. Maurer and M. Lener

When performing shoulder arthroscopy knowledge of the muscles, nerves and vessels lying in the vicinity of portals is important to prevent unnecessary complications.

Shoulder joint

The shoulder joint is a typical ball-and-socket joint and is protected by enveloping muscles. These muscles must be crossed when introducing the arthroscope and the necessary instruments.

Articular surfaces

As a classical ball-and-socket joint, the shoulder joint has a ball which is formed by the head of the humerus and a socket which is formed by the glenoid. The socket is not exactly perpendicular to the blade of the scapula, but has a physiological retroversion of 5°. The head of the humerus is separated from the shaft of the humerus by the anatomical neck. At the level of the greater tuberosity the cartilage covering of the articular surface has a recess which varies in size (Figs. 1 and 2).

The bony socket is formed by the glenoid cavity, narrowing superiorly, and has an anterior recess, the glenoid notch. The glenoid labrum enlarges the contact surface between the socket and the humeral head, which is 3 to 4 times larger. This articular lip is attached at the rim of the bony socket.

In section the glenoid labrum is triangular, approximately 4−6 mm thick at its base and 4 mm high from the base to the margin. It consists of a ring of collagen fiber bundles interspersed with fibrous cartilage in the surface facing the joint and at the base.

Except for one point at the anterior rim of the socket, the synovial layer of the joint capsule is attached to the glenoid labrum. This is the point where we may find the entrance to the subtendinous bursa of the subscapular muscle. Here, the articular lip is usually rather flat and protrudes freely into the joint cavity.

In the region of the supraglenoid tubercle the origin of the long head of the biceps is in continuity with the glenoid labrum. In the region of the infraglenoid tubercle the origin of the long head of the triceps is connected to the labrum.

Joint capsule

The capsule of the shoulder joint is slack with very weak ligaments, and is protected by a tendinous hood, the so-called rotator cuff (Fig. 4). The synovial membrane arises from the scapula at the free border of the glenoid labrum, except for the site where the joint space communicates ventrally with the subtendinous bursa of the subscapular muscle and where the attachment recedes to the base of the labrum. The fibrous membrane fuses with the outer surface of the glenoid labrum and radiates into the bone at its base. At the supraglenoid tubercle the fibrous capsule encloses the origin of the long head of the biceps brachii muscle. The capsule is attached to the humerus at its anatomical neck and only extends distally within the intertubercular sulcus. This is where the fibrous membrane, reinforced by fibers of the subscapular tendon, form the roof of the osteofibrous synovial canal in which the tendon of the long head of the biceps extends, surrounded by a 2–5 cm long tubular sheath (vagina synovialis intertubercularis).

When the arm hangs in its normal anatomical position the capsule is slack and forms the axillary recess, which disappears when lifting the arm.

Ligaments

The ligaments of the shoulder joint are very weak and consist of the glenohumeral ligaments, which are interwoven with the fibrous mebrane, and the coracohumeral ligament. The ventrally located glenohumeral ligaments are divided into the superior, middle and inferior glenohumeral ligaments. The opening of the subtendinous bursa of the subscapularis muscle lies between the superior and the middle glenohumeral ligaments. There is a recess in the region of the glenoid notch between the middle glenohumeral ligament and the glenoid labrum. The opening of the bursa, the middle glenohumeral ligament, as well as the subscapularis tendon can be readily viewed arthroscopically.

The coracohumeral ligament arises from the base of the coracoid process, radiates into the capsule and extends to the greater and lesser tuberosities.

Fornix of the humerus

The roof of the shoulder indirectly secures the shoulder joint and prevents the dislocation of the humeral head in a cranial direction (Fig. 5).

The fornix of the humerus is formed by the acromion, the coracoid process and the coracoacromial ligament which extends between both. The latter serves as a reinforcement at the point where the subdeltoid fascia and the supraspinatus fascia merge, and it generally has a triangular shape, the tip lying at the acromion. A lateral, stronger bundle of fibers extends from the undersurface of the acromion to the tip of the coracoid process and a medial, weaker bundle runs from the acromion to the base of the coracoid process. Occasionally this ligament is rectangular and then consists of parallel running fiber bundles.

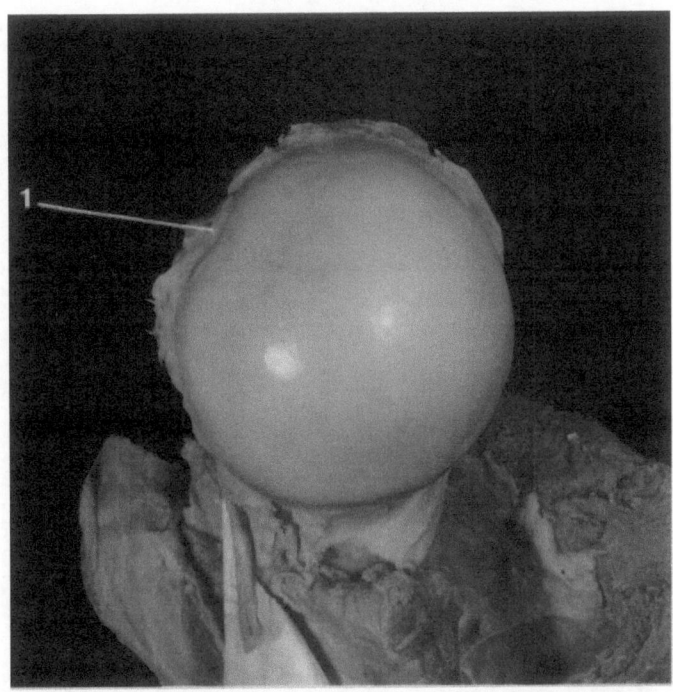

Fig. 1. Medial view of humeral head.
1 Area without cartilage

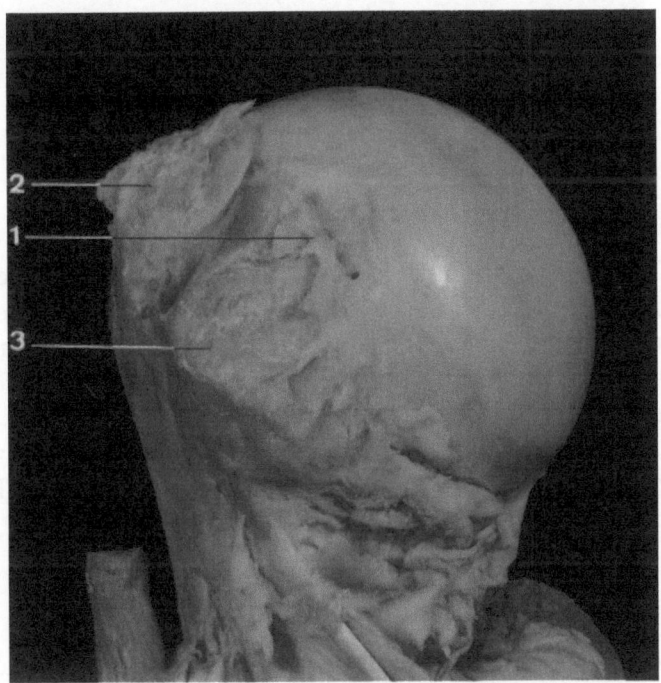

Fig. 2. Ventral view of humeral head.
1 Area without cartilage, *2* greater
tuberosity, *3* lesser tuberosity

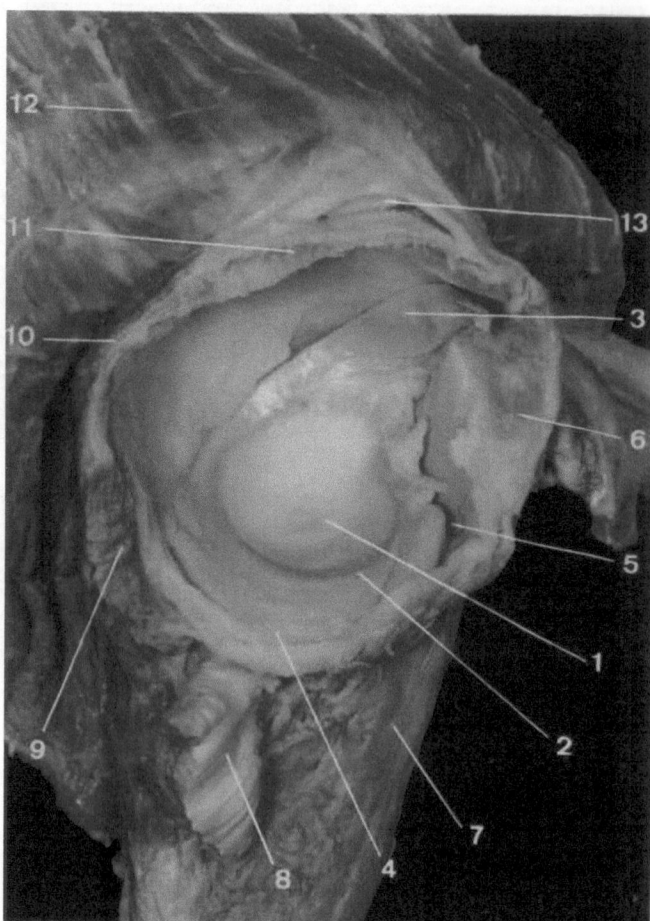

Fig. 3. Lateral view of shoulder joint (with humerus removed). *1* Glenoid cavity, *2* glenoid labrum, *3* long head of biceps brachii muscle, *4* axillary recess, *5* subtendinous bursa of the subscapularis muscle, *6* tendon of subscapularis muscle, *7* subscapularis muscle, *8* long head of triceps brachii muscle, *9* teres minor muscle, *10* infraspinatus muscle, *11* supraspinatus muscle, *12* deltoid muscle, *13* subacromial bursa

Joint cavity

The joint cavity is very spacious and has several recesses. The largest recess is formed anteriorly, connecting with the subtendinous bursa of the subscapularis muscle. Often it communicates with the subcoracoid bursa, thus further enlarging the joint cavity.

The synovial intertubercular sac is also one of the recesses of the joint cavity. The axillary recess is only evident with the arm by the side.

The joint cavity may be expanded to its maximum extent by filling it with fluid, thus making arthroscopy of the shoulder joint easier. It is also advisable to perform the arthroscopy when the arm is in mid-position.

Movements

Movements in the shoulder joint are possible around three main axes. From the neutral position, anteversion (flexion) and retroversion (extension) are performed around a trans-

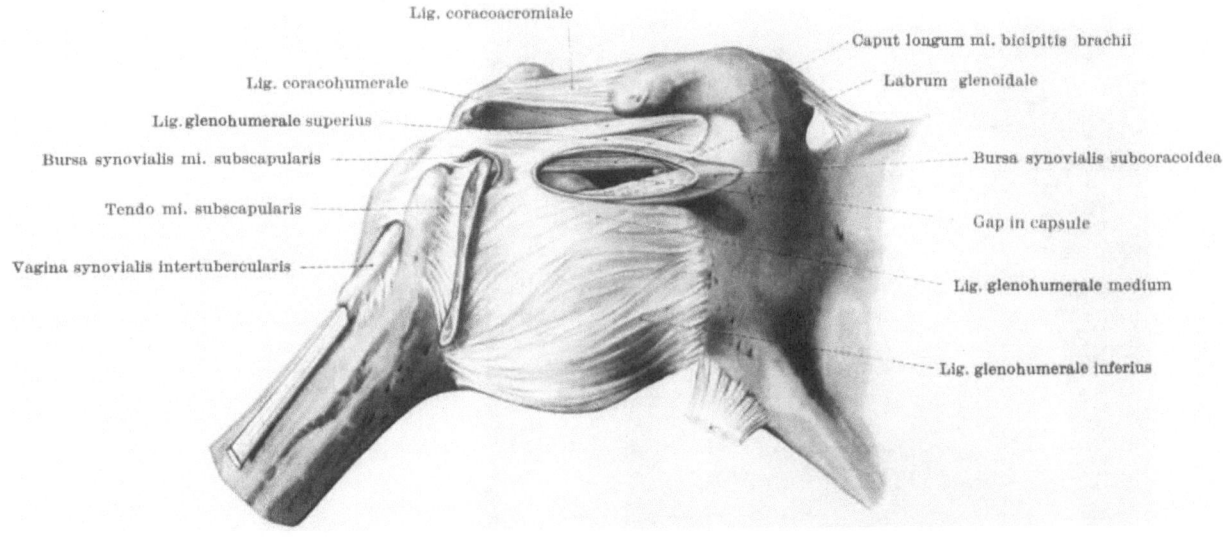

Lig. coracoacromiale

Caput longum mi. bicipitis brachii

Lig. coracohumerale

Labrum glenoidale

Lig. glenohumerale superius

Bursa synovialis mi. subscapularis

Bursa synovialis subcoracoidea

Tendo mi. subscapularis

Gap in capsule

Vagina synovialis intertubercularis

Lig. glenohumerale medium

Lig. glenohumerale inferius

Fig. 4. Neutral position of the shoulder joint (drawing from Lanz-Wachsmuth)

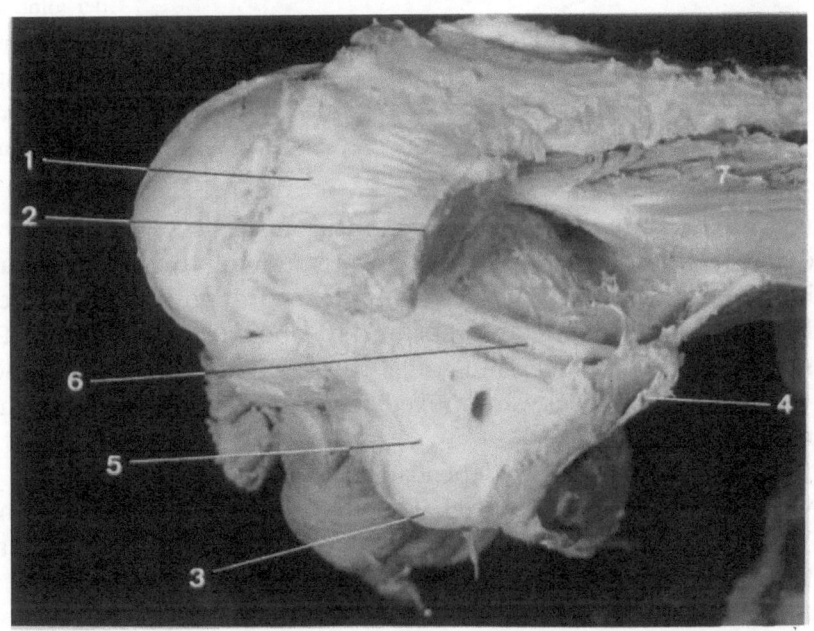

Fig. 5. Cranial view of fornix of humerus. *1* Acromion, *2* clavicular articular facet, *3* tip of the coracoid process, *4* coracoclavicular ligament (cut), *5* coracoacromial ligament (anterior fiber bundle), *6* coracoacromial ligament (posterior fiber bundle), *7* supraspinatus muscle

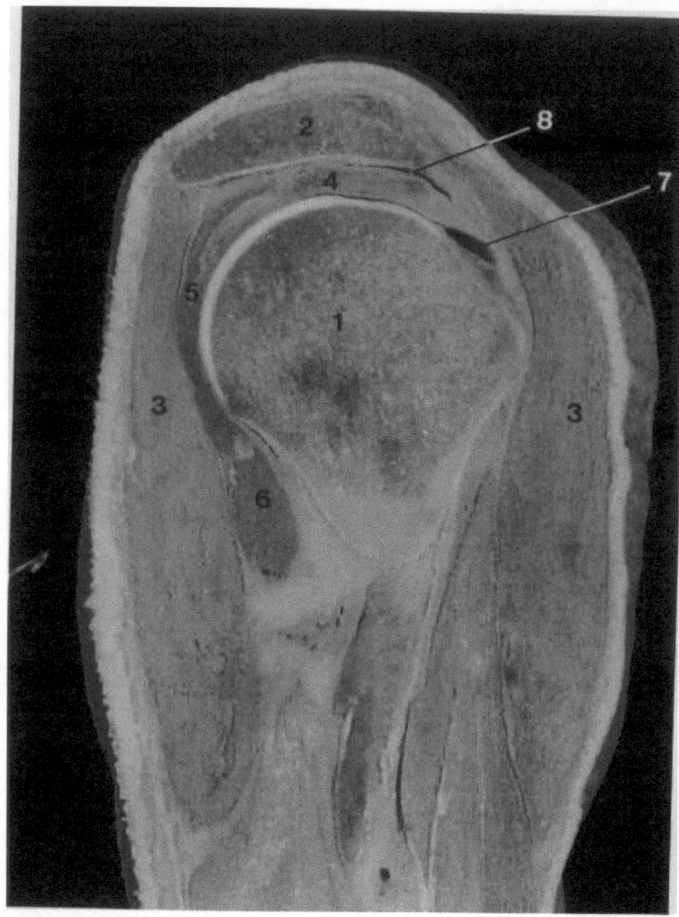

Fig. 6. Sagittal section through the shoulder joint. *1* Head of humerus, *2* acromion, *3* deltoid muscle, *4* supraspinatus muscle, *5* infraspinatuis muscle, *6* teres minor muscle, *7* intertubercular synovial sac, *8* subacromial bursa

verse axis, abduction and adduction around the sagittal axis of the scapula, and finally external and internal rotation on an axis running through the head and the capitulum of the humerus. Elevation of the arm from the neutral position is referred to as vertical movement. In the shoulder joint, anteversion and abduction are limited to approximately 90°, and retroversion to 40–50°. When the arm is slightly anteverted, adduction of 45° is possible.

Forward and backward movement with a 90° abduction of the arm is termed horizontal movement.

The range of rotation depends on the position of the shoulder joint and may be examined when the elbow joint is flexed. Thereby, additional rotation in the elbow joint is prevented. With the arm hanging by the side, internal rotation of up to 30° and external rotation of up to 60° is possible.

Rotator cuff

The shoulder joint is largely stabilized by the tone of the surrounding muscles. The tendons of these muscles enclose the head of the humerus superiorly, anteriorly and posteriorly, thus

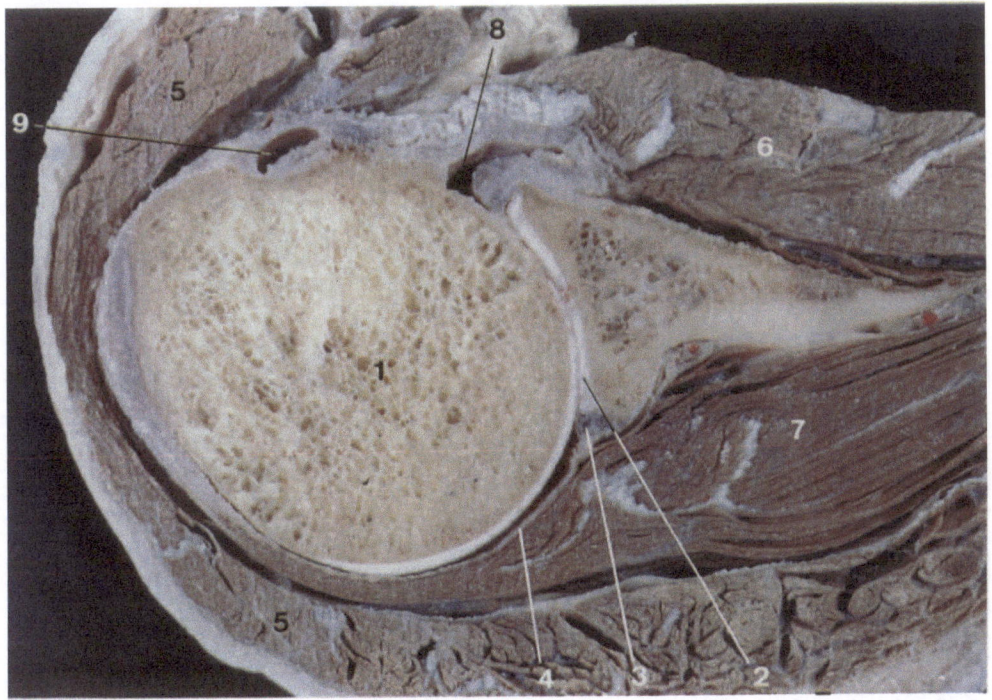

Fig. 7. Transverse section through the shoulder joint. *1* Head of humerus, *2* glenoid cavity, *3* glenoid labrum, *4* articular capsule, *5* deltoid muscle, *6* subscapularis muscle, *7* infraspinatus muscle, *8* subtendinous bursa of subscapularis muscle, *9* intertubercular synovial sac

forming a tendon hood which covers three quarters of the joint capsule. The tendon hood is fused with the capsule, thereby preventing the formation of folds and incarceration of the capsule. Additional stability is provided by the overlying muscle belly of the deltoid and the long head of the biceps tendon, which runs through the joint cavity and passes over the humeral head (Fig. 6).

The bursae of the subacromial and subdeltoid spaces are of considerable importance for rotator cuff function. In particular, they aid movement of the supraspinatus tendon, as it passes through a constriction between the fornix of the humerus and the proximal end of the humerus when leaving the osteofibrous space of the supraspinous fossa.

Pathological changes in this region can result in pain on abduction ("painful arc"). Ruptures of the tendon usually lead to tears in the joint capsule and the synovium.

Supraspinatus muscle

The supraspinatus muscle is completely covered by other muscles. Its origin in the supraspinous fossa and fascia lies deep to the trapezius muscle. Its tendon passes below the fornix of the humerus and the deltoid muscle, where it then becomes fused superiorly with the shoulder joint capsule, to reach the upper facet of the greater tuberosity of the humerus.

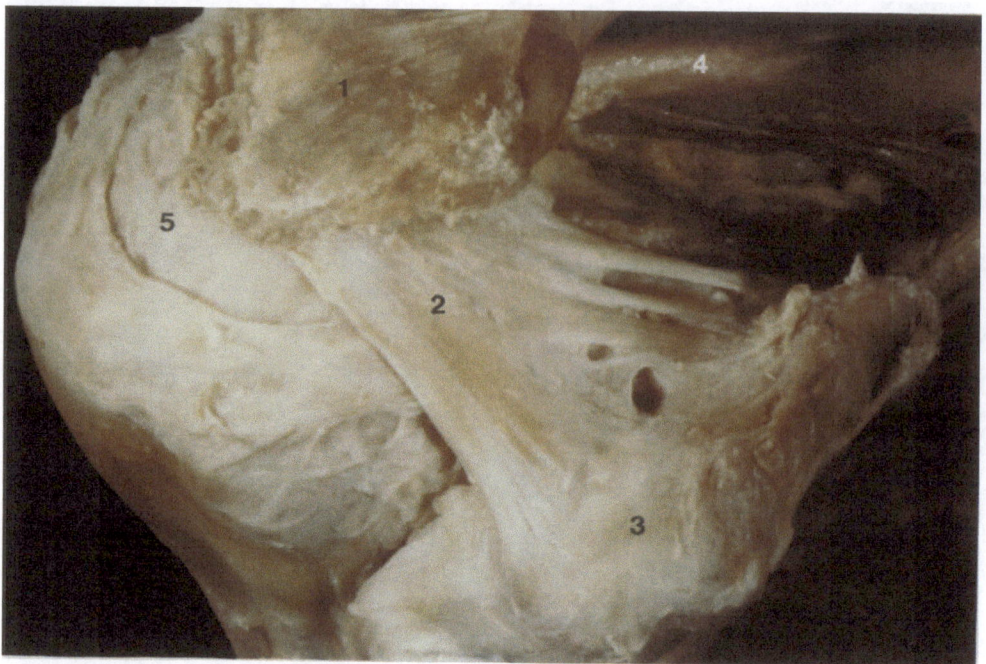

Fig. 8. Cranial view of subacromial synovial space. *1* Acromion, *2* coracoacromial ligament, *3* coracoid process, *4* supraspinatus muscle, *5* subacromial bursa (opened cranially)

The supraspinatus muscle is an abductor, a capsule tensor and a guiding muscle in the shoulder joint. When abducting the arm, the deltoid muscle pulls the greater tuberosity under the fornix of the humerus. Rotation of the humerus displaces the supraspinatus tendon. External rotation positions it under the acromion and internal rotation positions it under the coracoacromial ligament.

The supraspinatus muscle is supplied by the suprascapularis nerve.

Infraspinatus muscle

This muscle arises from the infraspinous fossa and fascia, leaving space for the neurovascular bundle of the suprascapular nerve and vessels at the neck of the scapula. Covered by the posterior part of the deltoid, which in part arises from the infraspinous fascia, the infraspinatus muscle, fuses dorsally with the joint capsule and inserts into the middle facet of the greater tuberosity. The upper surface of the tendon is covered by the subacromial bursa. The main function of the infraspinatus muscle is external rotation but its lower fibers also contribute to adduction. It is innervated by the axillary nerve.

Teres minor muscle

This muscle arises from the lateral margin of the scapula, superior to the origin of the teres major and inserts on the lower facet of the greater tuberosity. Its tendon strengthens the joint

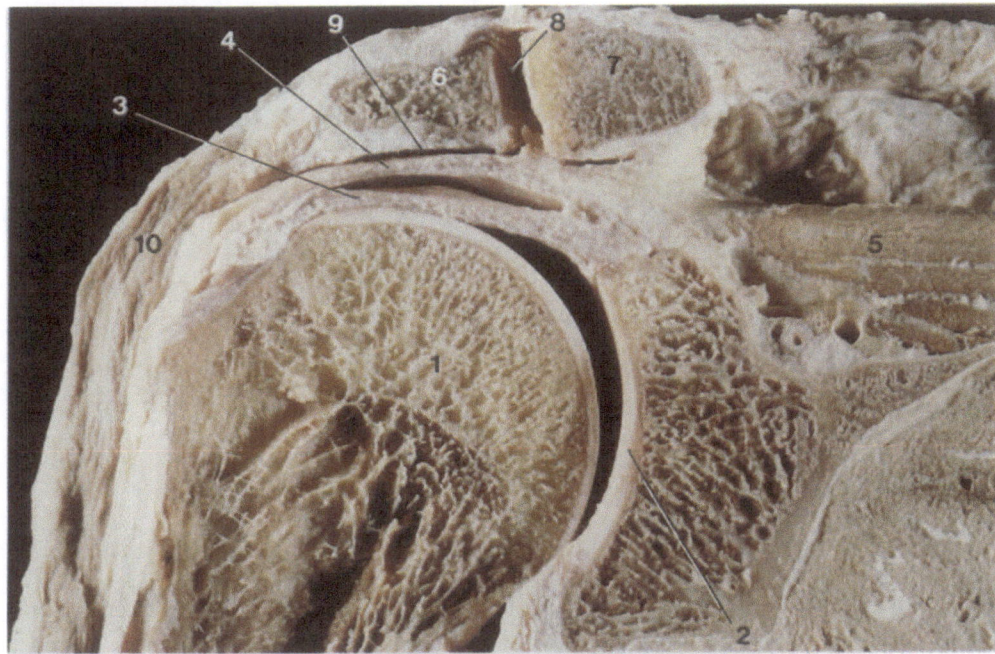

Fig. 9. Frontal section through the shoulder joint. *1* Head of humerus, *2* glenoid cavity, *3* long head of biceps brachii muscle, *4* joint capsule with supraspinatus tendon radiating into it, *5* supraspinatus muscle, *6* acromion, *7* clavicle, *8* acromioclavicular joint, *9* subacromial bursa, *10* acromial part of deltoid muscle

capsule posteriorly and inferiorly. The teres minor acts as an external rotator of the arm contributes to adduction. Is innervated by the subscapular nerve.

Subscapularis muscle

This muscle arises in the subscapular fossa. Its tendon passes anteriorly to the shoulder joint and inserts into the lesser tuberosity and the proximal part of its crest. Some of its fibers pass over the intertubercular sulcus and reach the crest of the greater tuberosity. The subscapularis tendon is fused with the anterior surface of the joint capsule, thereby strengthening it (Fig. 7).

The subtendinous bursa of the subscapularis muscle lies between the subscapularis tendon and the neck of the scapula. It communicates with the glenohumeral joint and often also with the subcoracoid bursa. The upper margin of the tendon protrudes freely into the bursa.

The subscapularis is a strong internal rotator and its cranial fibers participate in abduction. It is supplied by the subscapularis nerve.

Deltoid muscle

The three sections of this muscle take origin from the lateral one-third of the clavicle (clavicular part), the acromion (acromial part) and the spine of the scapula (scapular part). All three parts insert into the deltoid tuberosity on the lateral aspect of the humeral shaft.

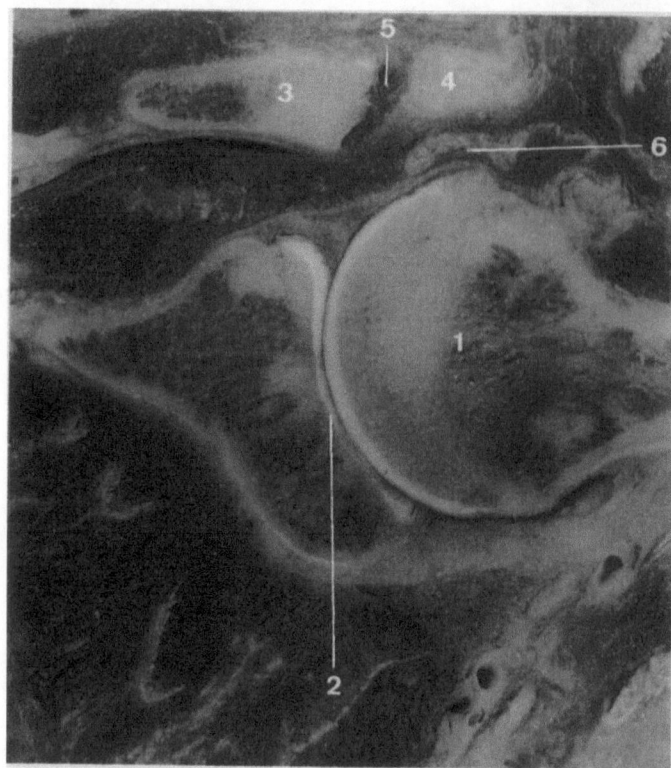

Fig. 10. Frontal section through the shoulder joint with abducted arm. *1* Head of humerus, *2* glenoid cavity, *3* clavicle, *4* acromion, *5* acromioclavicular joint, *6* supraspinatus muscle in the subacromial space

The three parts of the muscle differ in function depending on the relative position of the shoulder joint and the muscle fibers to the axes of movement. The acromial part of the deltoid muscle is the most important abductor of the shoulder joint. This function cannot be replaced by the other abductors. When abducting over 60°, the action of the acromial part is assisted by the other two parts, which are normally active in adduction. The clavicular part effects anteversion and internal rotation. The spinal part helps with retroversion and external rotation. The deltoid muscle plays a major role in all movements of the shoulder joint, thus indirectly stabilizing the joint. Innervation is supplied by the axillary nerve.

Biceps brachii muscle

The long head of this muscle takes its origin from the supraglenoid tubercle and from the glenoid labrum which is intracapsular. At the level of the deltoid tuberosity it joins with the short head arising from the coracoid process. The biceps brachii muscle has two insertions. The deep insertion is into the radial tuberosity, whereas the superficial insertion is into the bicipital aponeurosis, passing medially into the antebrachial fascia. With its long head the biceps acts as an abductor and internal rotator, whilst the short head aids adduction and anteversion of the shoulder joint. At the elbow joint the function of the biceps is flexion and, in the flexed position, it also acts as a strong supinator of the forearm. Innervation is supplied by the musculocutaneous nerve.

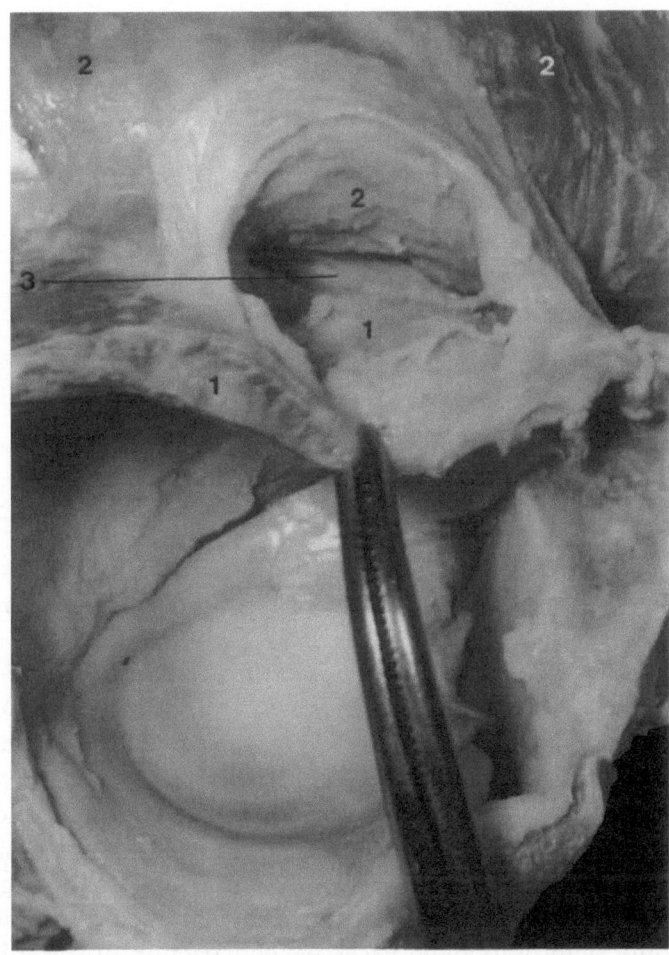

Fig. 11. Lateral view of subdeltoid bursa and subacromial bursa (communicating). *1* Tendon of supraspinatus muscle (floor of bursa), *2* deltoid muscle (roof of bursa), *3* coracoacromial ligament (roof of bursa)

The tendon of the long head plays an important role in arthroscopy of the shoulder joint because of its location within the joint space. Surrounded by a synovial membrane, the tendon passes over the humeral head to the intertubercular sulcus in which it continues distally, enclosed by the intertubercular synovial sac. When the arm is rotated internally, tension of the tendon decreases, whereas in external rotation, tension increases.

Subacromial space

The narrow osseofibrous space between the fornix of the humerus and the subdeltoid space on the one hand, and the proximal end of the humerus and the joint capsule on the other, contains the supraspinatus tendon and the cranial part of the infraspinatus tendon (Fig. 8).

When abducting the arm from the neutral position, the greater tuberosity is pulled under the fornix of the humerus by the supraspinatus muscle, and the tendons mentioned above are

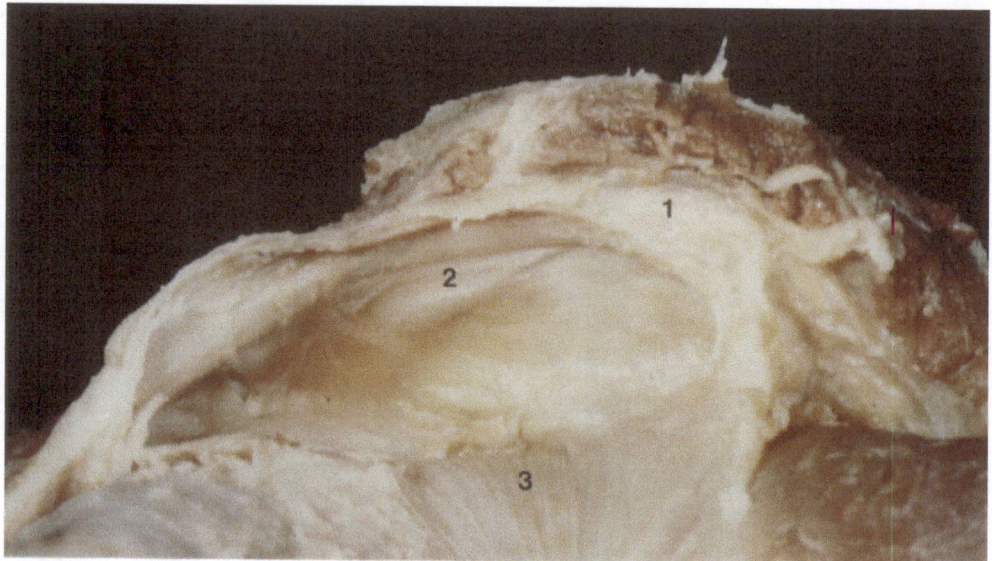

Fig. 12. Lateral view of subacromial bursa (with deltoid muscle removed). *1* Acromion, *2* coracoacromial ligament, *3* supraspinatus tendon

protected by the subacromial and the subdeltoid bursae. The two bursae are usually connected with each other (Figs. 9 and 10).

The roof of the two bursae is formed by the deltoid muscle, the coracoacromial ligament and the acromion. The upper surface of the supraspinatus tendon lies in the floor. Pathological changes in this region cause pain when abducting the arm up to 120° (Figs. 11 and 12).

The subacromial space can be examined by bursoscopy. The arm should be abducted only slightly to avoid excessive constriction of the subacromial space. Pathological changes in this region may lead to the development of additional articular surfaces on the undersurface of the acromion.

Relationships to nerves and vessels

To protect the neurovascular structures of the axilla the arm should be only moderately abducted (Figs. 13 and 14).

In marked abduction, the axillary vessels and the infraclavicular part of the brachial plexus are under tension and may be damaged if the anterior portal is made too far medially and/or inferiorly with the musculocutaneous nerve being especially vulnerable.

If the posterior portal is located too far inferiorly, the axillary nerve may be damaged. Lesions of nerves and vessels can be avoided if the portals are located correctly.

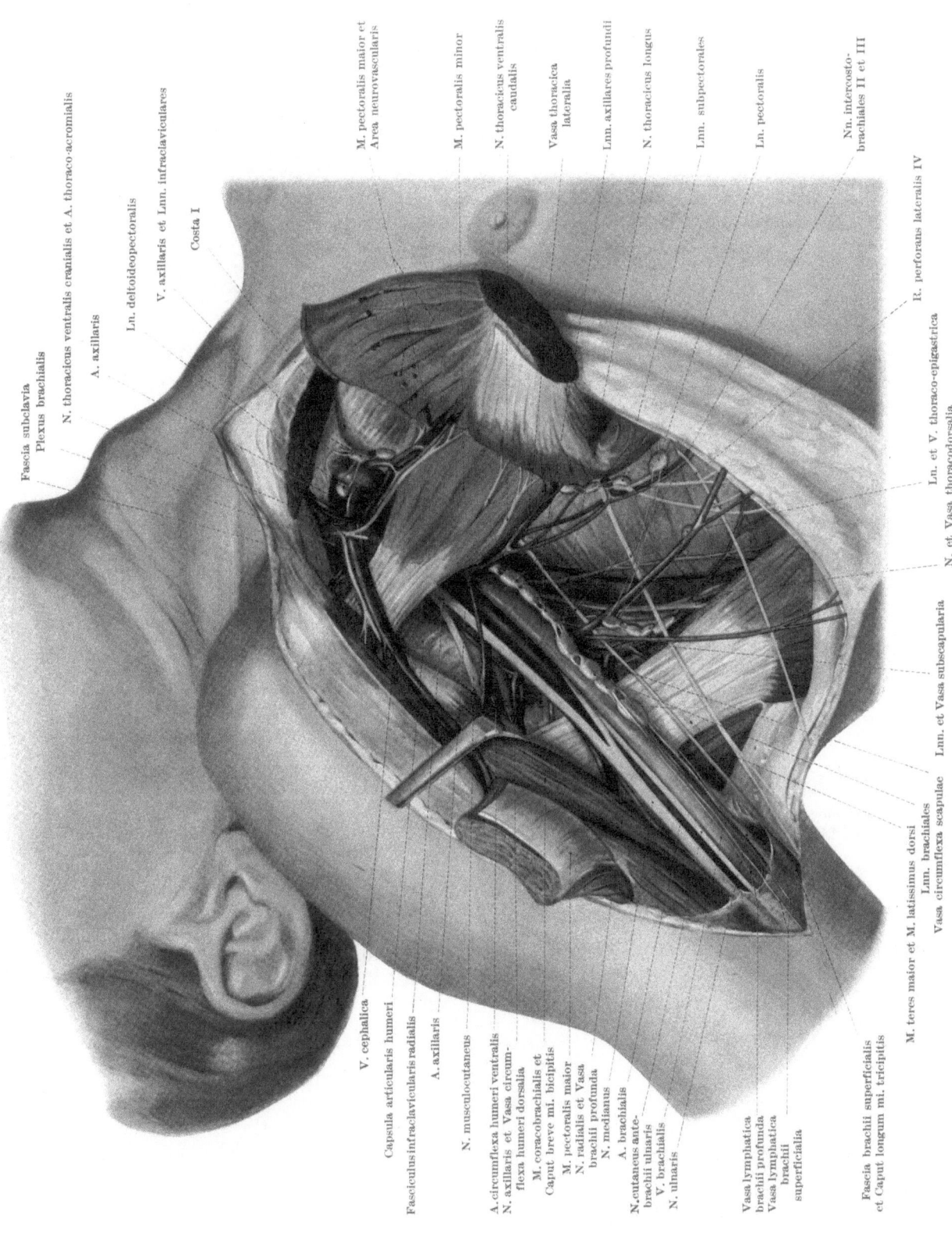

Fig. 13. Topography of the axilla (drawing from Lanz-Wachsmuth)

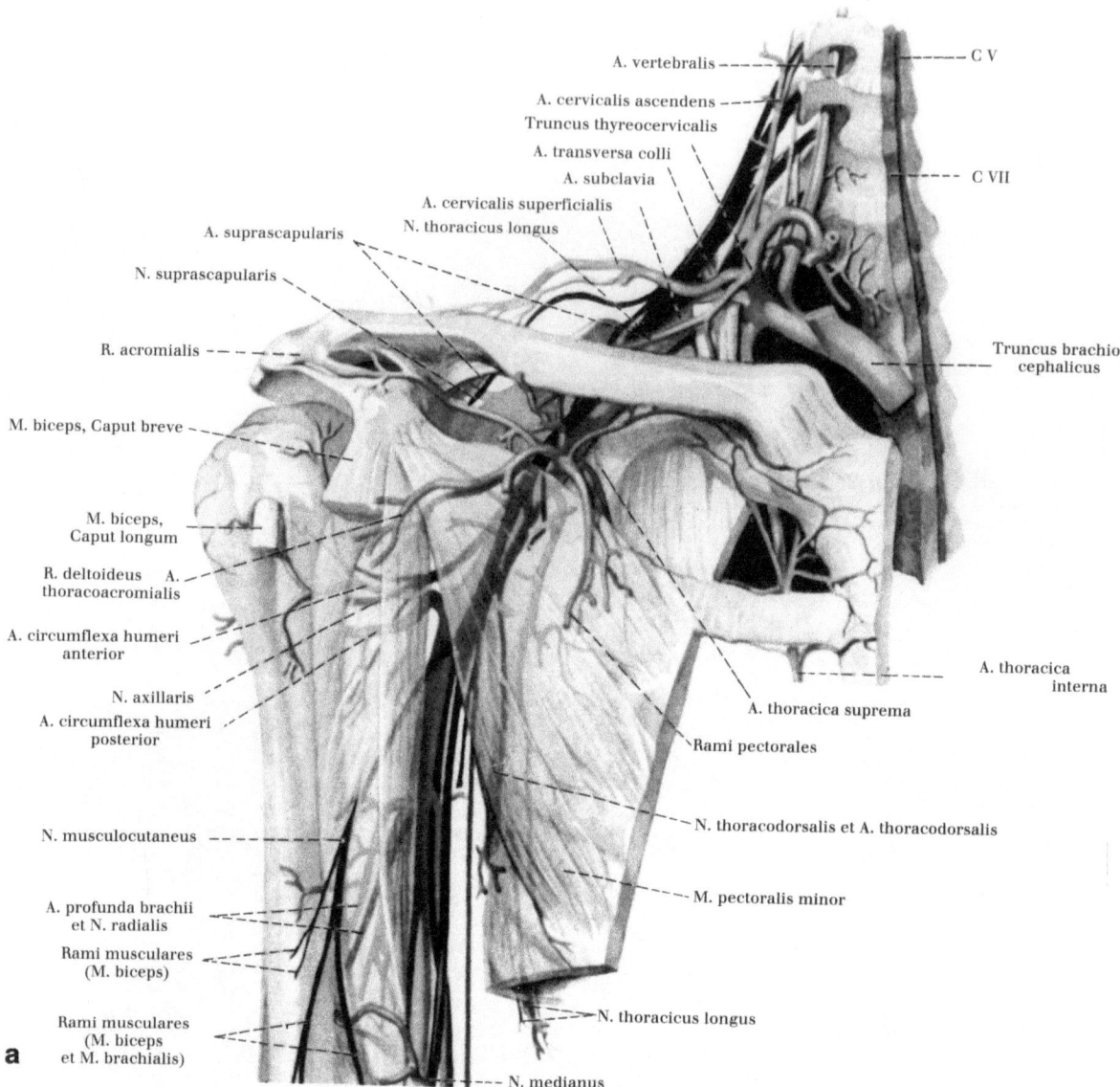

A. vertebralis
A. cervicalis ascendens
Truncus thyreocervicalis
A. transversa colli
A. subclavia
A. cervicalis superficialis
N. thoracicus longus

A. suprascapularis
N. suprascapularis
R. acromialis
M. biceps, Caput breve
M. biceps, Caput longum
R. deltoideus   A. thoracoacromialis
A. circumflexa humeri anterior
N. axillaris
A. circumflexa humeri posterior
N. musculocutaneus
A. profunda brachii et N. radialis
Rami musculares (M. biceps)
Rami musculares (M. biceps et M. brachialis)

a

C V
C VII
Truncus brachio cephalicus
A. thoracica interna
A. thoracica suprema
Rami pectorales
N. thoracodorsalis et A. thoracodorsalis
M. pectoralis minor
N. thoracicus longus
N. medianus

Fig. 14. Survey of the nerves and vessels of the shoulder (drawing from Braus-Elze)

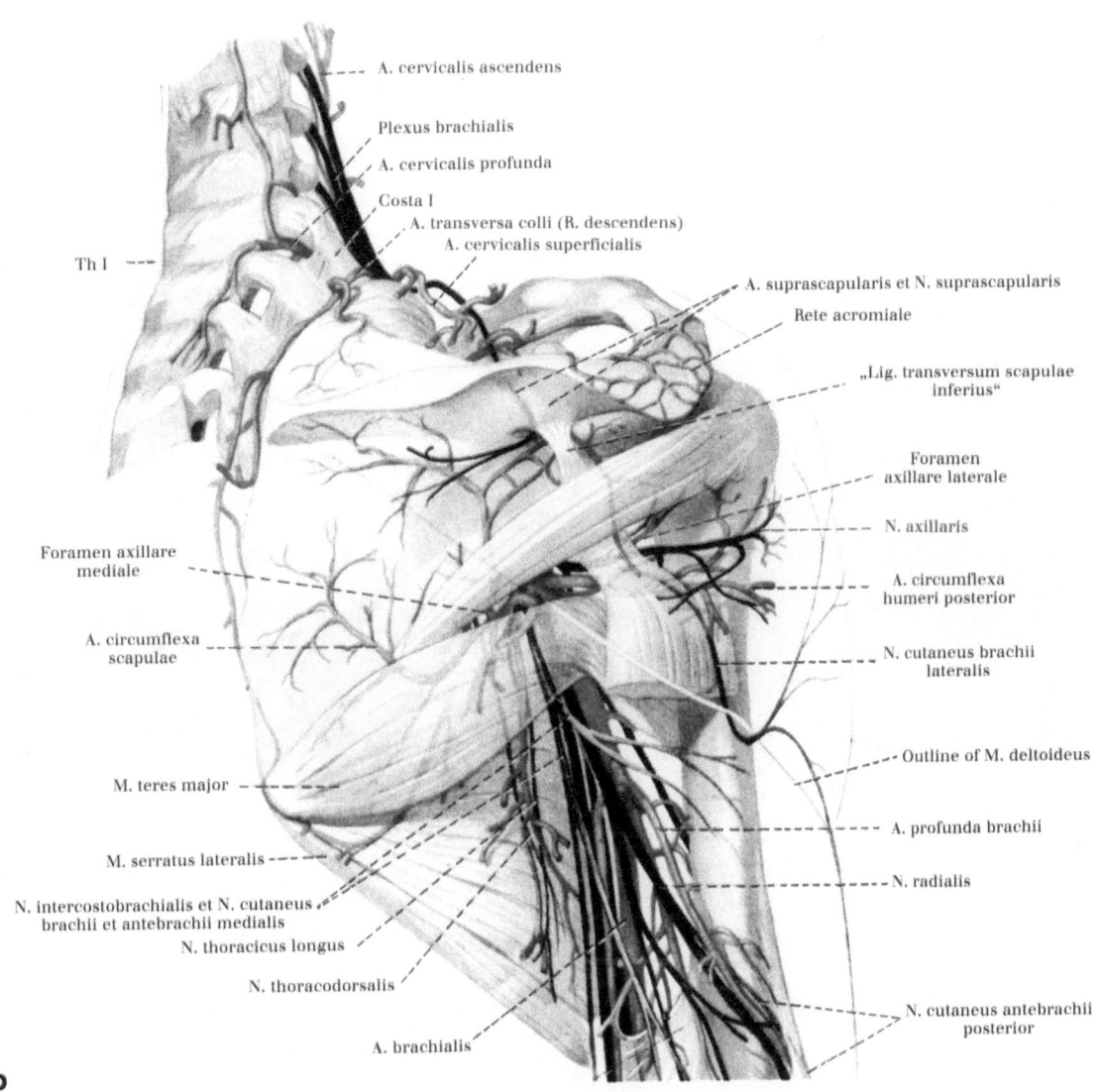

A. cervicalis ascendens

Plexus brachialis

A. cervicalis profunda

Costa I

A. transversa colli (R. descendens)
A. cervicalis superficialis

Th I

A. suprascapularis et N. suprascapularis

Rete acromiale

„Lig. transversum scapulae inferius"

Foramen axillare laterale

N. axillaris

Foramen axillare mediale

A. circumflexa humeri posterior

A. circumflexa scapulae

N. cutaneus brachii lateralis

Outline of M. deltoideus

M. teres major

A. profunda brachii

M. serratus lateralis

N. radialis

N. intercostobrachialis et N. cutaneus brachii et antebrachii medialis

N. thoracicus longus

N. thoracodorsalis

A. brachialis

N. cutaneus antebrachii posterior

b

Innervation of the skin

Anteriorly, superiorly and laterally the skin of the shoulder is innervated by the supraclavicular nerves of the cervical plexus. The lateral superior cutaneous branch of the axillary nerve innervates the so called "badge area" laterally. Posteriorly, the region supplied by the dorsal branches of the spinal nerves may extend to the area of the posterior approach. This can be important during regional anesthesia, as a brachial plexus block may not produce complete anesthesia posteriorly.

2 Anesthesia for shoulder surgery

I. Braito, R. Habeler, and H. Resch

Operative interventions in the shoulder are very demanding with regard to anesthetic requirements. In particular, problems may result from the following.

- proximity of the operative area to the face, necessitating special draping techniques,
- special positioning and the possible consequences on the circulation,
- particular requirements with regard to the quality of vision in arthroscopic interventions,
- preexisting concomitant illness of the patient.

Depending on the kind of shoulder surgery performed, general anesthesia or regional anesthesia may be employed for the actual operative intervention [1]. Another consideration is postoperative analgesia, usually as important for the patient as the intraoperative analgesia. More advanced techniques of regional anesthesia have distinct advantages over the conventional postoperative treatment with strong analgesics and their associated unwanted side effects [2].

General anesthesia

Preoperative assessment is performed as in other elective surgery. The patients are examined one day prior to the operation on the ward or in the anesthesia outpatient department by an anesthetist. The most appropriate anesthetic technique is chosen after consideration of anesthetic problems as well as aspects of operative technique. The patient's wishes for a specific anesthetic procedure should, of course, be taken into account. One hour prior to the operation premedication is routinely administered with an opiate drug and atropine given intramuscularly. Before placing the patient in the half-sitting position, which has proven to have negative effects on the circulation, 500 ml of a crystalloid solution are infused in order to counteract possible hypotension. If general anesthesia is used, it should be in the form of a balanced anesthesia, as insufflation anesthesia with mechanically supported ventilation. The tubing and the anesthetic equiment should be placed contralateral to the operative area in order to avoid disconnections or kinking of the tube if the patient's position needs to be changed intraoperatively. Mechanical ventilation as well as positioning for the operation generally require complete muscular relaxation of the patient [2].

Special care and attention is required from the anesthetist when surgery is completed. Application of the dressing and manipulation of the shoulder may lead to coughing and unpredictable defensive movements in the lightly anesthetized patient. More so than in other surgery, these unwanted movements may put a strain on the surgical wound and jeopardize the success of the intervention.

Advantages:
– swift start of the operation,
– 100% success rate,
– even a long procedure creates minimal discomfort for the patient.
Disadvantages:
– circulatory instability related to special positioning
– end-phase of anesthesia problematic
– short postoperative analgesia

Regional anesthesia

If regional anesthesia (Figs. 15 and 16) has been agreed upon with the patient, premedication can be dispensed with in most cases. For operations in the shoulder, interscalene plexus block as described by Winnie is very suitable [3, 5, 6]. In this procedure the nerve fibres of the brachial plexus are blocked at their passage through the scalene interval. The point of passage is found at the level of the cricoid, at the posterior margin of the sternocleidomastoid muscle. The needle is inserted in a medial-posterior-inferior direction. Depending on the body weight, 15 to 30 ml of a local anesthetic agent are used. The extent of the block usually includes the segments C4 to C8, sometimes T1 is also involved. This method generally provides excellent analgesia for interventions in the shoulder. Our experience with this technique has been satisfactory in nearly 90% of the cases. For operations at the anterior-inferior glenoid rim (e.g., Bankart procedures) where the sensory segments T1 and T2 are present, plexus blocking according to Winnie's technique is not always suitable. These problematic segments (intercostobrachial nerves) either require a supplementary intercostal block T1 and T2 (beware pneumothorax!) or induction of a supplementary local anesthesia in the margin of the operative area by the surgeon.

The combined use of a quick-acting (lidocaine 2%) with a long-lasting local anesthetic (bupivacaine 0.5%) ensures good operative conditions with regard to positioning, relaxation and application of bandages as well as a postoperative analgesia effect of about 7 hours. One particular advantage of this procedure is the possibility of prolonged local anesthesia postoperatively by means of a catheter. Due to the high patient acceptance rate, this technique is ideally suited to provide postoperative pain relief whilst allowing early mobilization (Fig. 17). For this purpose a local anesthetic is administered 3 times a day in the form of a bolus (e.g., 10 to 15 ml bupivacaine 0.25%) [3].

Side effects and complications:
– Temporary, relatively insignificant side effects (e.g., Horner's syndrome) occur with varied frequency. Complications are rare (e.g., paresis of the phrenic nerve). In contrast to the supraclavicular anesthesia of the plexus, pneumothorax or lesions to the nerves are very infrequent.

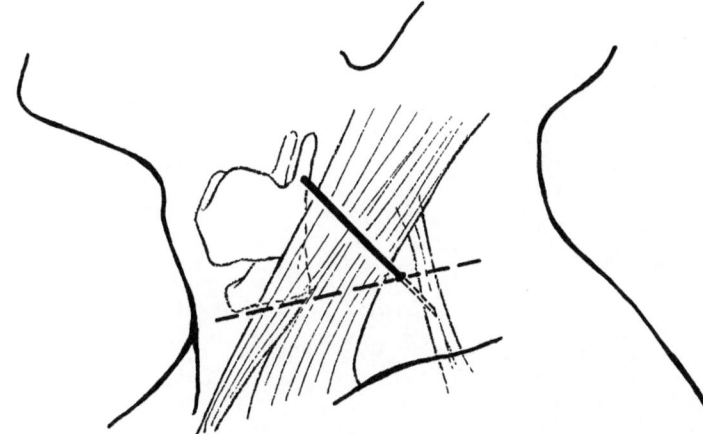

Fig. 15. Interscalene plexus block; Introduction of the needle on the posterior edge of the sternocleidomastoid muscle at the level of the cricoid; the needle is directed dorsomedially

-   Serious incidents (puncture of the peridural or subarachnoidal space) have been described as rarities in literature, however, they may be largely avoided if the prescribed direction of injection is adhered to [4].

Contraindications:
-   Contralateral injuries and/or concomitant thoracic procedures,
-   insufficient patient compliance, or rejection of this method by the patient.

Advantages:
-   excellent intra- and postoperative analgesia,
-   no circulatory instability,
-   high rate of patient acceptance in procedures of short duration.

Disadvantages:
-   more time-consuming anesthesia,
-   longer duration of operation affects patient,
-   difficult anesthetic conditions when the block is insufficient or wearing off.

Anesthetic problems in arthroscopic surgery

Suboptimal visual conditions in shoulder arthroscopy are often due to excessive bleeding, especially if the duration of the operation is long. It is often difficult to improve, even with thorough irrigation. Rather than jeopardizing the surgery, undesired bleeding can be minimized by preventing hypertension or even reducing the mean arterial pressure (MAP) to 70–80 mm Hg.

Once an increase in blood pressure due to pain or insufficient sedation of the patient has been excluded, drug induced hypotension (MAP 50–60 mm Hg) may become necessary in the rare case if the bleeding cannot be otherwise controlled. This kind of anesthesia, which affects the autoregulation mechanisms of the patient considerably, should only be employed in the patients of the ASA group 1, that is to say in those patients without any recognizable organic illness. If difficult operative conditions are expected, the possibility of intraoperative controlled hypotension should have been scheduled prior to the operation by the surgeon and

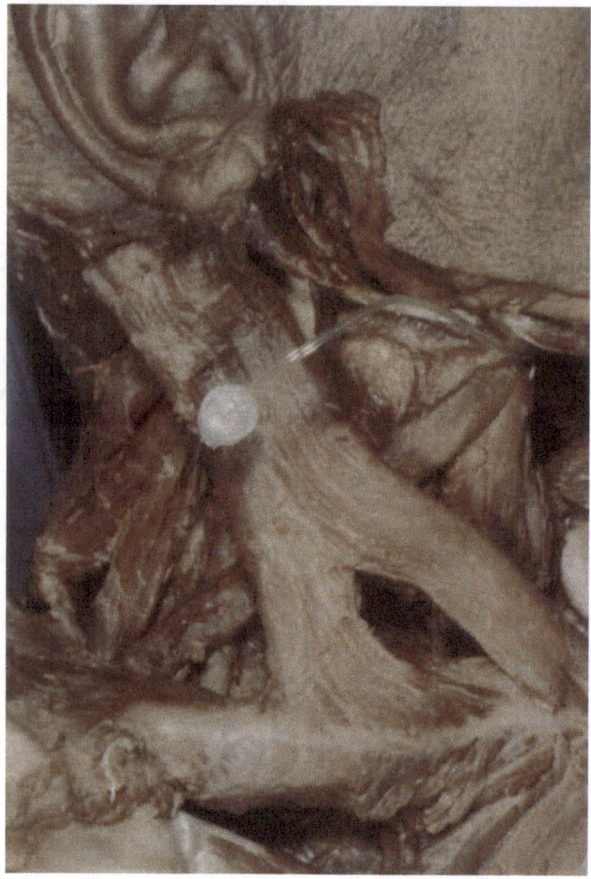

Fig. 16. Anatomical specimen; tip of the block needle is placed in the scalene interval (where the omohyoid muscle and the anterior scalene muscle cross)

the anesthetist. Thus a detailed examination and preparation of the patient as well as comprehensive planning of anesthesia maximizes the success of the operation. The pharmacological principle of the method, varying with the drugs used, is based on a dilatation of the terminal venous and/or arterial branches of the vascular system with subsequent reduction of the blood pressure. A decrease in blood pressure below critical values may lead to insufficient perfusion in the capillary regions of sensitive organs (e.g., brain, liver, kidney), causing profound organic lesions or intensifying them. A thorough preliminary examination is thus as essential as is detailed intraoperative monitoring of blood pressure and kidney function as well as blood gases and acid/base balance. Postoperatively, after discontinuing the hypotensive drugs, close monitoring is required due to the possible hypertensive rebound of the circulation (beware of postoperative hemorrhage).

Short-acting, low toxicity and easily controllable substances should be used for controlled hypotension. Of the drugs available at present (sodium nitroprusside and other nitroprepa-rations, calcium antagonists, alpha- and beta receptor blockers) none meets all these require-ments.

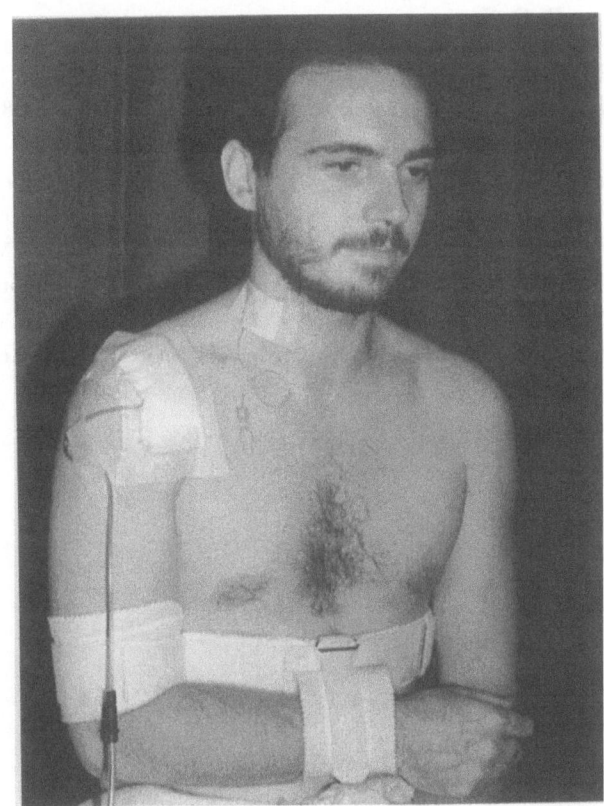

Fig. 17. Patient after operation with the arm immobilized; catheter for prolonged postoperative anesthesia to ensure postoperative pain relief and painless early motion

The combination of locally employed vasoconstrictors (injection of epinephrine solutions, vasopressin, etc.) with controlled hypotension does not seem useful as both procedures are based on a contradictory pharmacological principle. Overdosage, increased absorption or accidental intravascular injection can lead to systemic reactions such as blood pressure crises, vegegative phenomena, and hyperperistalsis during general anesthesia. The anesthetist and the surgeon should therefore discuss and plan the anesthetic procedure and the management of a possible intraoperative bleeding prior to surgery.

All in all, the relatively demanding procedure of controlled hypotension is only very rarely employed, as sufficient anesthesia and the subsequent slight reduction of the MAP usually ensure adequate control of unwanted bleeding.

References

1. Cadoret J (1984) Anesthesia in surgery of the shoulder. Soins Chir 36:15−18
2. Conn RA, Cofield RH, Byer DE, Linstromberg JW (1987) Interscalene block anesthesia for shoulder surgery. Clin Orthop 216:94−98
3. Van Laack W, Hennes A, Refisch A (1987) Mobilization of the partially stiff shoulder under anesthesia (ankylosing humero-scapular periarthritis). Clin Orthop 125:669−673
4. Vester-Andersen T, Christiansen C, Hansen A, Sörensen M, Meisler C (1981) Interscalene brachial plexus block: area of analgesia, complications and blood concentrations of local anesthetics. Acta Anaesth Scand 25:81−85
5. Ward ME (1970) The interscalene approach to brachial plexus. Anesthesia 29:147−151
6. Winnie AP (1970) Interscalene brachial plexus block. Anesth Analg 49:455−458

3 Preparation for arthroscopy

K. Golser, H. Resch, and M. Lener

Arthroscopy of the glenohumeral joint and bursoscopy of the subacromial space are becoming increasingly important for both establishing a diagnosis and, in particular, for the treatment of the injuries and diseases of the shoulder joint. Careful physical examination and assessment by modern imaging techniques provide for accurate diagnosis and may indicate the need for arthroscopic intervention. Purely diagnostic arthroscopy can be performed on an outpatient basis, especially when regional anesthesia is used. In this case all patients undergo thorough medical examination at our own anesthesia outpatient department prior to the operation. This helps to keep the incidence of complications to a minimum. For shoulder arthroscopic surgery we find it helpful to standardize positioning, draping and instrumentation in order to guarantee a smooth procedure.

Indications

Shoulder arthroscopy should be regarded as supplementary to other techniques in the assessment of shoulder pain. It should not be used routinely as the preferred diagnostic aid. Arthroscopy and bursoscopy are only indicated after appropriate preoperative assessment. The indications for shoulder arthroscopy are only briefly summarized here; the following chapters contain more detailed descriptions.

Possible indications for arthroscopy of the glenohumeral joint:
- recurrent subluxation of the shoulder,
- recurrent dislocation of the shoulder with uncertain direction of the dislocation or inadequate CT evaluation,
- multidirectional instability,
- fresh bony Bankart lesion,
- frozen shoulder,
- suspected S.L.A.P. lesion,
- shoulder pain of uncertain etiology, refractory to treatment.

Indications for bursoscopy and subacromial decompression:
- impingement syndrome, refractory to conservative management,
- impingement syndrome with radiologically demonstrated subacromial osteophytes,
- incomplete rotator cuff tears,

– calcific tendinitis, refractory to treatment,
– subacromial debridement in cases of large irreparable rotator cuff tears.

Anesthesia

The anesthetic possibilities will be reviewed in short and explained from a surgical viewpoint. Arthroscopic interventions can in principle be carried out under general or regional anesthesia. Scalene block, described in detail in Chap. 2, can be used for almost all arthroscopic surgery in the shoulder, provided that the anesthetist is sufficiently experienced. General anesthesia with ventilation allows the systemic blood pressure to be decreased and thus bleeding to be controlled. The difference in pressure (systolic blood pressure – irrigation fluid pressure in the subacromial space) should not amount to more than 50 mm Hg. A mean arterial pressure of approx. 80 mm Hg provides the optimal circumstances for good vision in the subacromial space (see Chap. 7).

When using regional anesthesia, controlled reduction of blood pressure is not possible. Therefore, the subacromial space, and in particular the area of the acromial branch of the thoracoacromial artery at the end of the acromion, should be infiltrated with approximately 2 ml POR 8 (ornithine-vasopressin diluted in 20 ml NaCl) to provide for local vasoconstriction. The greater part is injected into the subacromial space to provide for inflation and vasoconstriction. With the exception of bursoscopy, scalene block must be regarded as the anesthetic procedure of choice when performing shoulder arthroscopy, as the systemic effects are minimal, positioning is simplified, and there is the benefit of postoperative analgesia.

Positioning

The patient can be placed in the lateral recumbent position or in a half-sitting position, the so-called "beach-chair" position.

Lateral recumbent position

The upper part of the body is stabilized by flexible padded supports. A foam rubber wedge is placed between the patient's legs to ensure a comfortable position (especially important under regional anesthesia) and to prevent pressure sores. The upper body is inclined 30° posteriorly, which positions the socket of the shoulder joint in the horizontal plane [7] (Fig. 18). This position facilitates the handling of the instruments and allows for the adjustment of the angle in case of a possible labral reattachment. The patient's arm is stabilized with the elbow joint at a right angle in a specially designed arthroscopic elbow brace (Gell, Innsbruck), (Fig. 19). This brace consists of right-angled gutters, made of plastic, which can be fixed with velcro straps (Fig. 20). Good padding of the soft tissues, particularly the posterior aspect of the ulna, with surgical wool is imperative in order to avoid pressure sores. A multidirectional swivel table can be positioned over the patient's chest for instruments (Fig. 21). In line with the axis of the humeral shaft a traction device is attached to the plastic support. Via a pulley the shoulder is distracted with 3–4 kg for arthroscopy and 5–6 kg for bursoscopy, with the humeral shaft in 30 to 40° of abduction. Less traction is required for

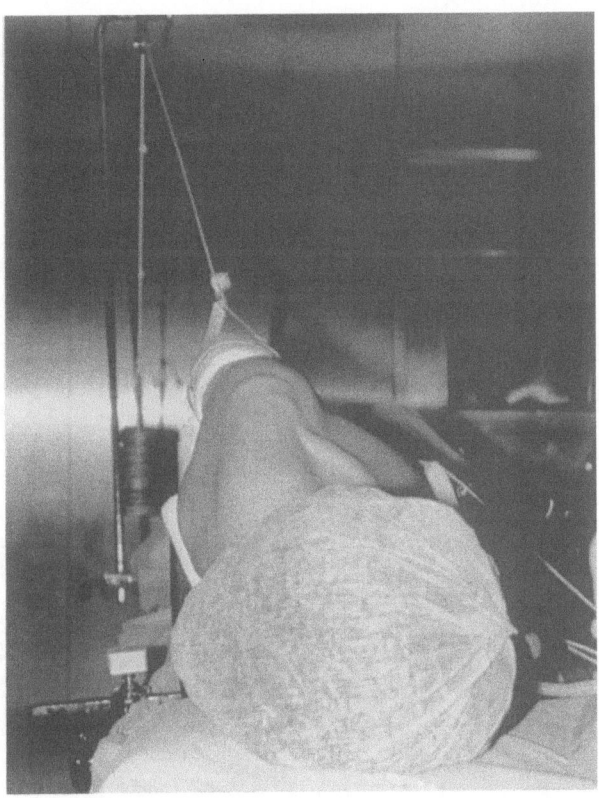

Fig. 18. Lateral recumbent position – upper part of the body in 30° posterior inclination

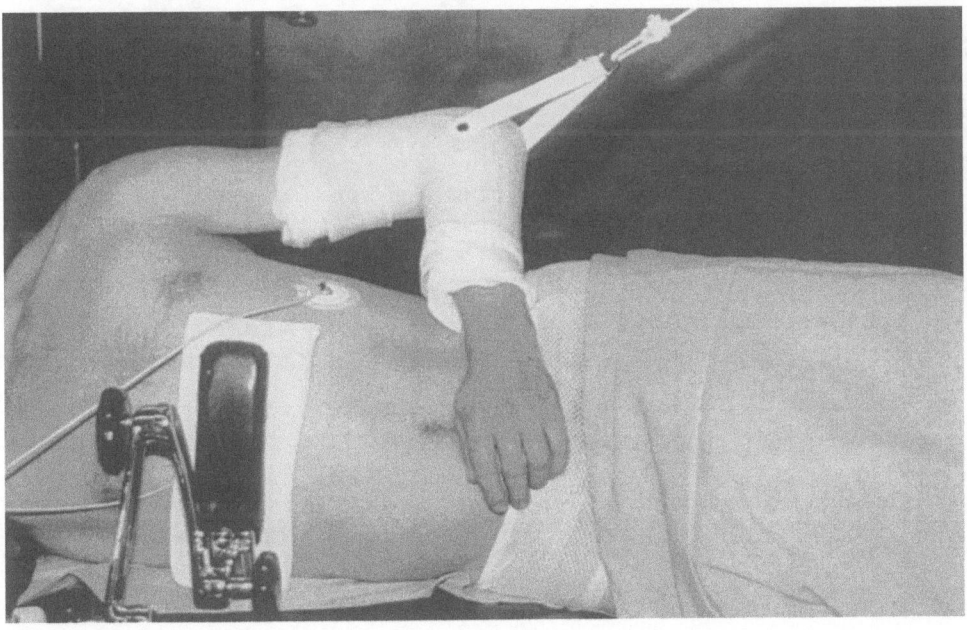

Fig. 19. Arm placed in elbow brace with traction device. Upper part of body stabilized by flexible, padded support

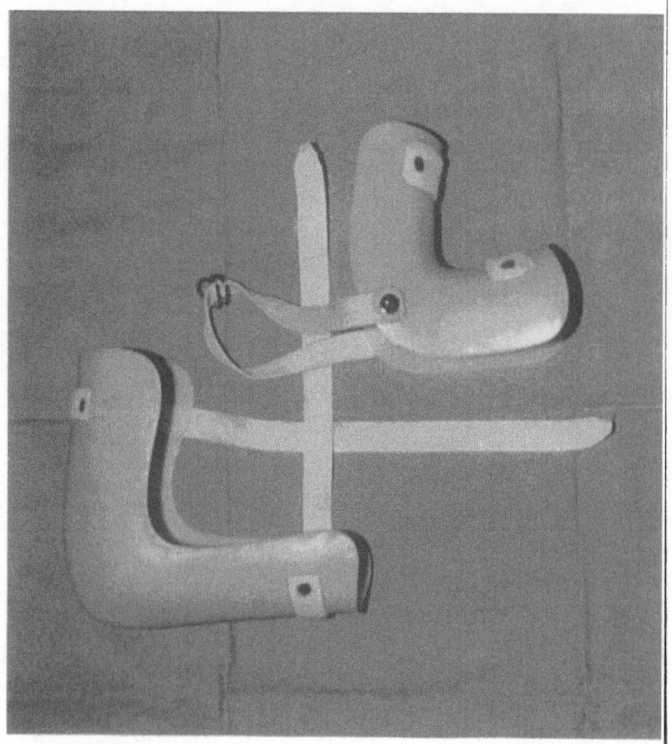

Fig. 20. Arthroscopic elbow brace
(according to Resch)

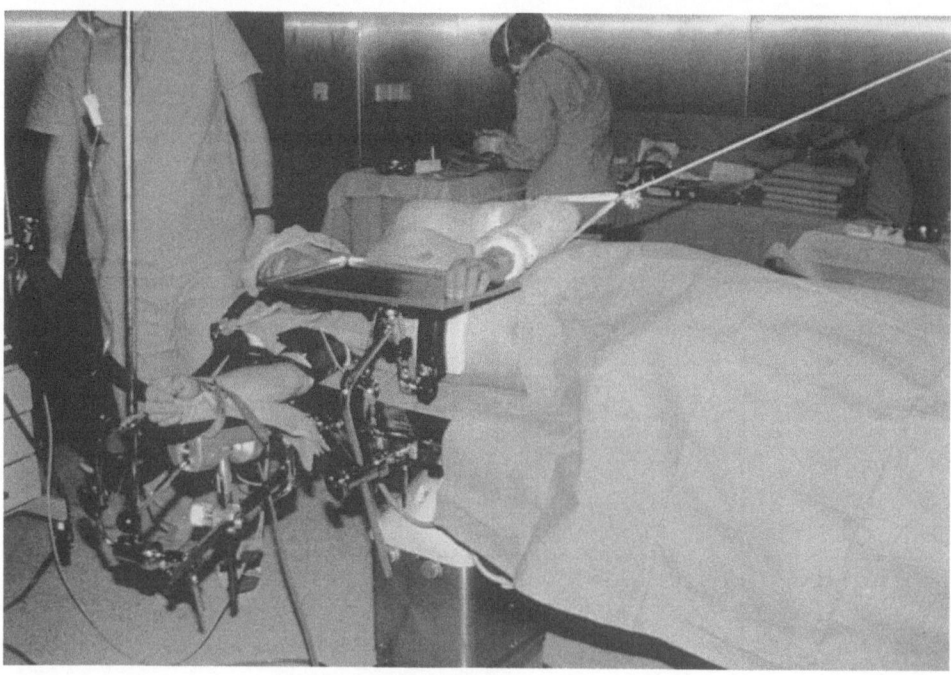

Fig. 21. Patient in lateral recumbent position with multidirectional swivel table for instruments

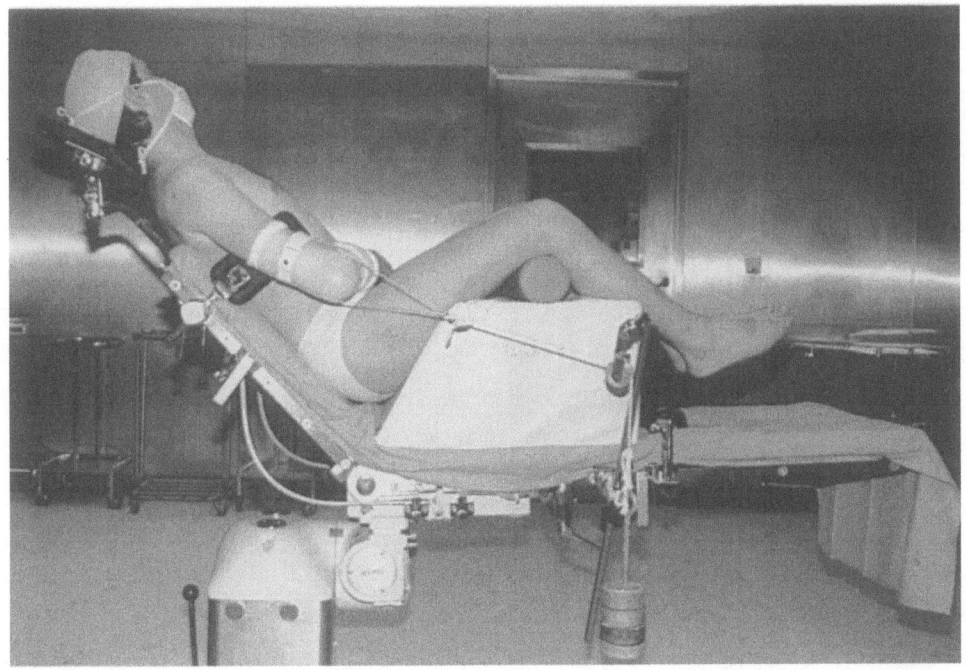

Fig. 22. Half-sitting position ("beach-chair" position)

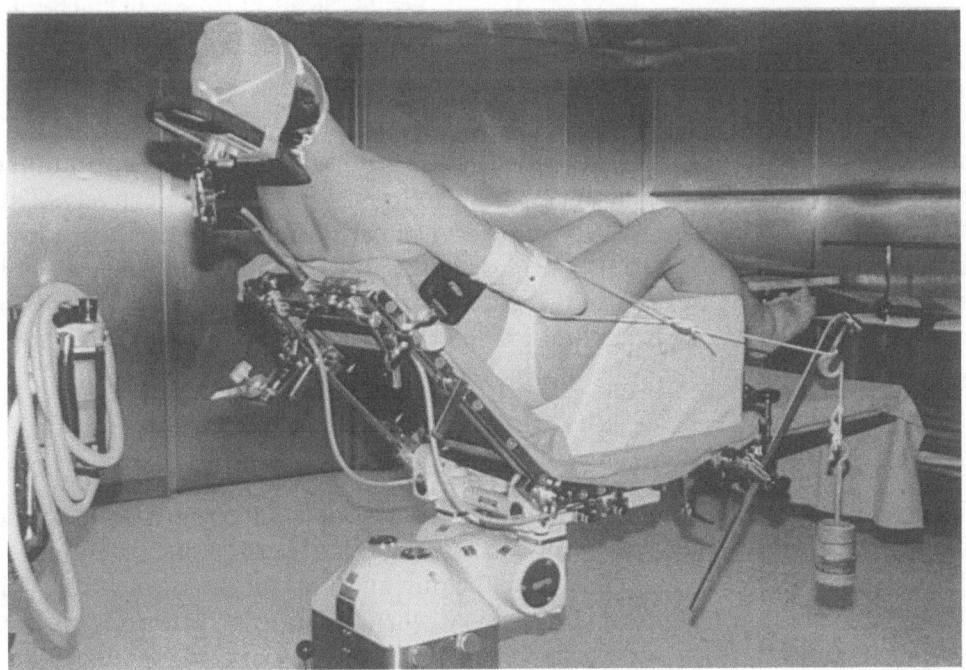

Fig. 23. Half-sitting position. Posterior view. The whole shoulder readily accessible

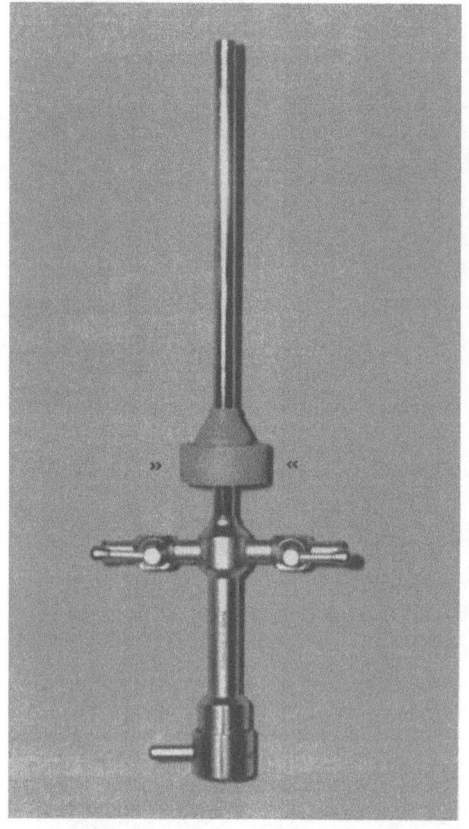

Fig. 24. Sheath of scope with "rubber diaphragm" as seal against back flow of irrigation fluid

small or female patients. This special arm brace allows for controlled rotation of the humeral head and for the capsule and ligament structures to be tensed selectively. Thus, careful and functional inspection of these structures can be performed during arthroscopy. With this arm brace the rotator cuff can also be inspected and palpated more thoroughly during bursoscopy. Positioning of the arm is most important when performing an arthroscopic labrum reattachment. Unless an exact and predetermined degree of external rotation is used during reattachment, mobility can be unnecessarily restricted postoperatively.

Half-sitting position ("beach-chair" position)

This position [9] is an alternative to the lateral recumbent position, and we now tend to use it almost exclusively. The patient sits on a 30 cm thick foam rubber cushion, so that the whole shoulder and scapula is situated above the outer edge of the operating table (Figs. 22 and 23). This elevated sitting position is necessary when performing a limbus suture, as the whole scapula should be freely accessible. The upper body is elevated 50–60° from the horizontal and is stabilized laterally with a flexible support slightly below the axilla. The arm is held in 30–40° of abduction via a pulley. The traction weight can be reduced by 2–3 kg as compared

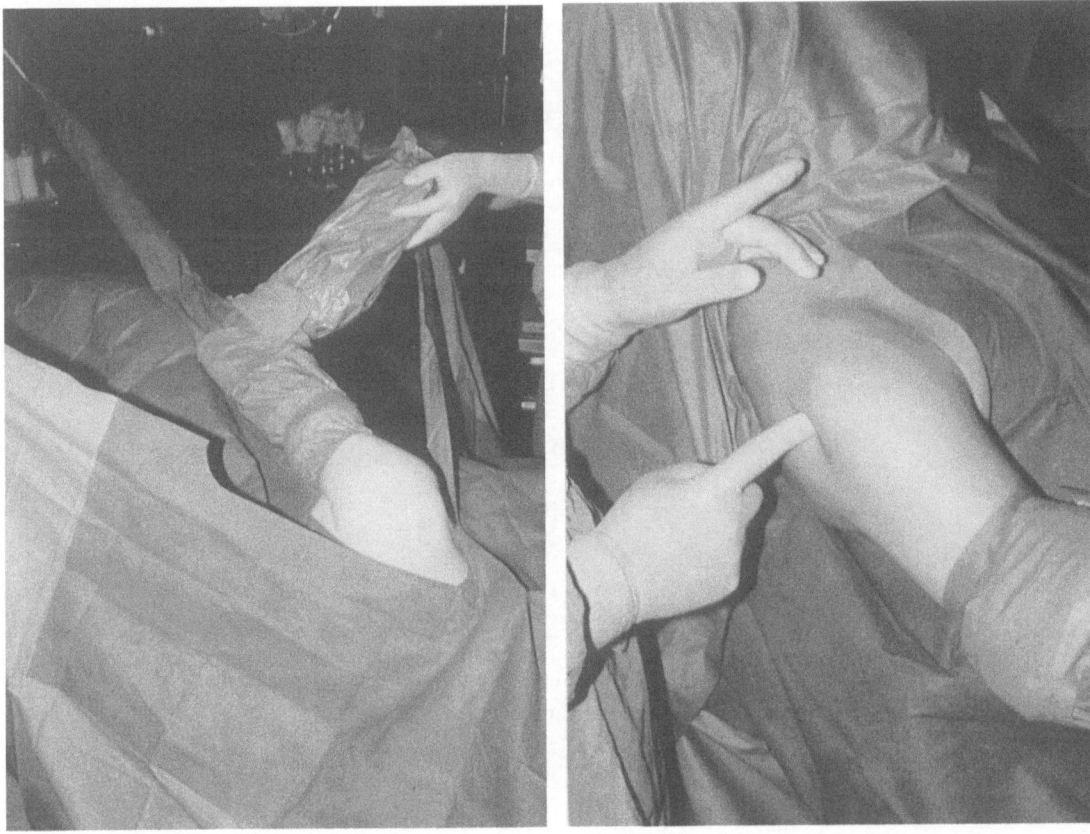

Fig. 25   Fig. 26

Fig. 25. Waterproof sterile draping with arm free

Fig. 26. Half-sitting position. Patient with waterproof draping, palpation of the posterior portal

to the lateral recumbent position since traction against gravity is not required. Patients undergoing arthroscopy under regional anesthesia find this position to be very comfortable. The beach-chair position also has several advantages for the surgeon and therefore it is an excellent alternative to the lateral recumbent position:

– open surgery can be performed subsequently, if necessary, without changing the patient's position.
– orientation for handling of instruments is facilitated (especially advantageous for the setting of the drill direction at limbus reattachment).
– the patient is not affected by the irrigation fluid if the draping leaks.

The only major drawback of this position is the descending position of the arthroscope. Water flowing down along the sheath may enter the camera and blur the picture. This technical complication can be avoided by slipping a rubber diaphragm, taken from a "Universal Cannula" (Acufex), on to the sheath (Altcheck; see also Chap. 6) (Fig. 24).

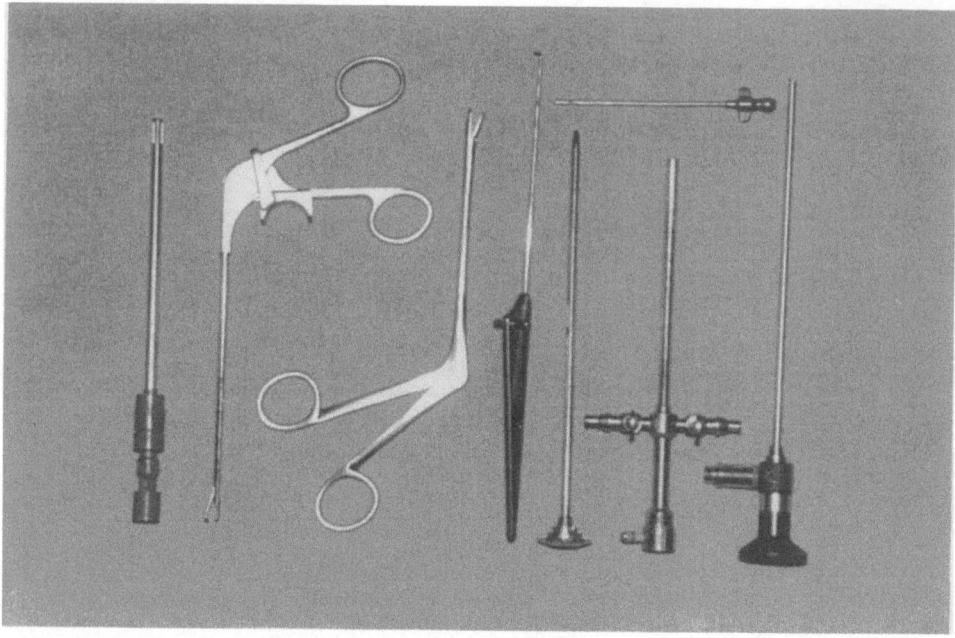

Fig. 27. Standard instrumentation. From left to right: synovial resector, pit bull, rongeur, probe, blunt trocar, arthroscopic sheath, 30° wide-angle scope, Cushing cannula (transverse placement)

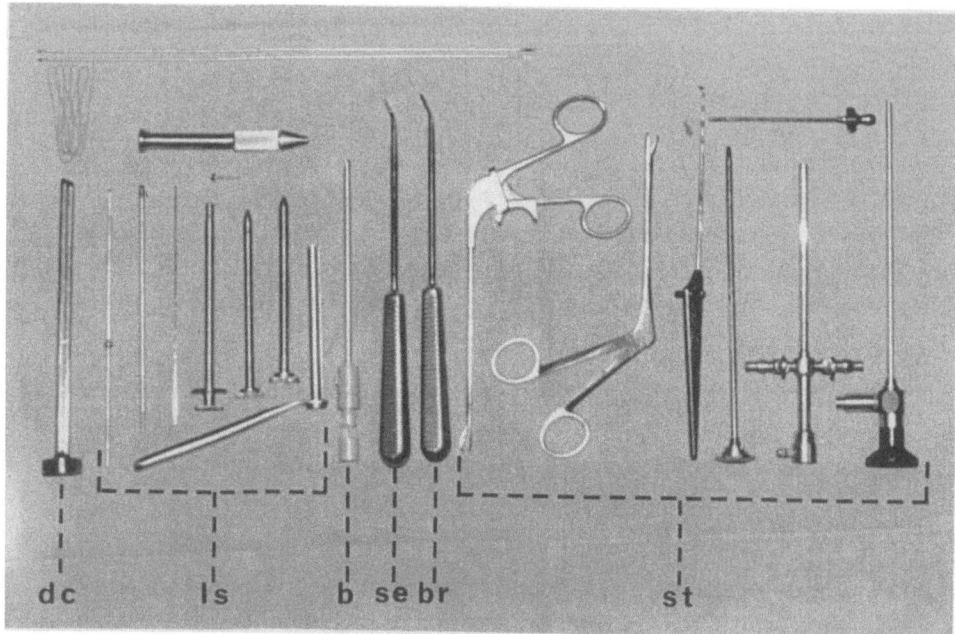

Fig. 28. *dc* Double-lumen cannula, *ls* labrum screw fixation set (transverse placement of handle), *b* burr with ball tip (arthroplasty burr), *se* shoulder elevator, *br* Bankart rasp, *st* standard instrumentation

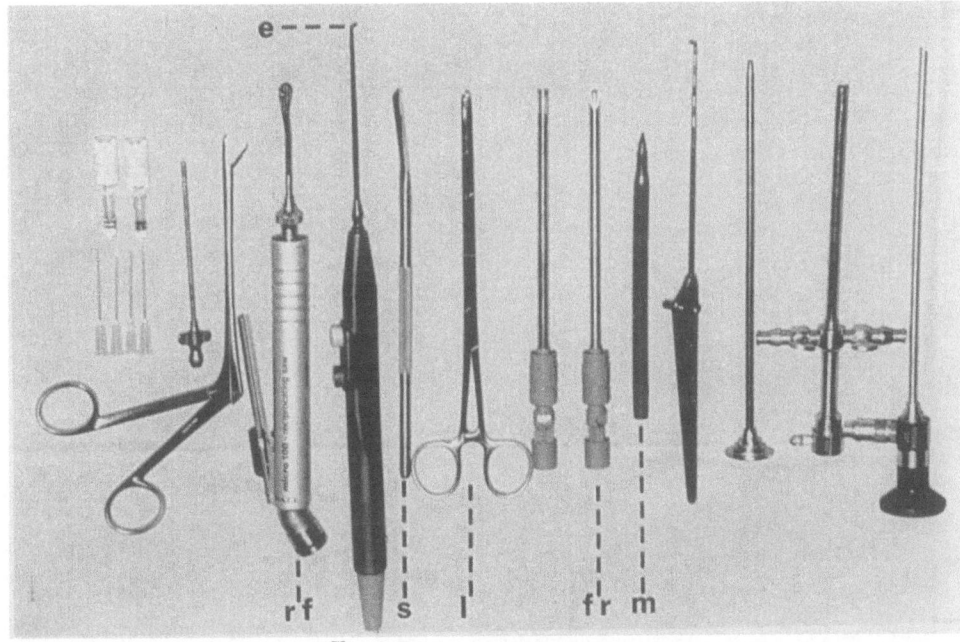

Fig. 29. *rf* Reciprocating file, *e* electrosurgical knife, *s* sliding knife, *l* ligament forceps, *fr* full-radius resector, *m* marking pencil

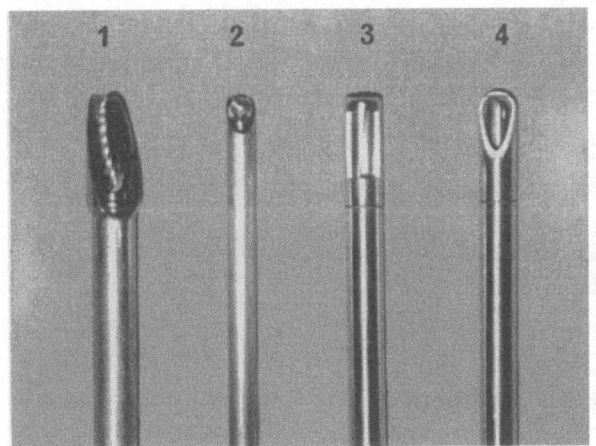

Fig. 30. Shaver attachments. *1* Acromionizer, *2* arthroplasty burr, *3* synovial resector, *4* full-radius resector

The irrigation fluid normally used is Ringer's lactate. If bursoscopic surgery is planned, use of the electrosurgical knife requires the electrolyte solution to be substituted with a sugar solution (Resectal). If there is no possibility of reducing the systemic blood pressure, a controlled increase in the irrigation fluid pressure is invaluable. This can be achieved by hanging the fluid bag extremely high (ceiling attachment) or by using a pressure controlled pump system.

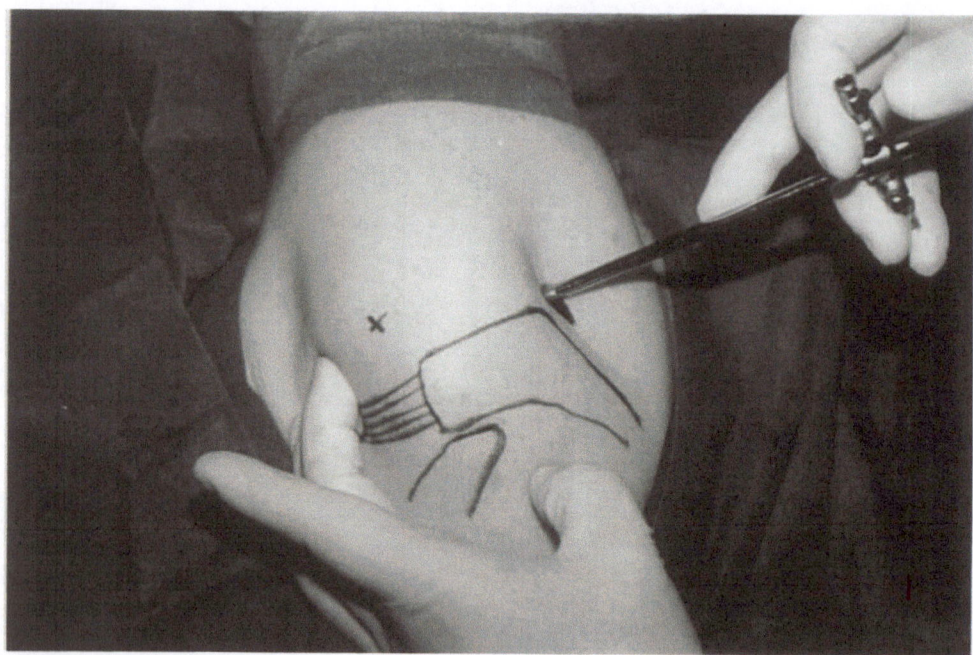

Fig. 31. Introduction of sheath of scope through posterior portal. Lateral view, patient in beach-chair position

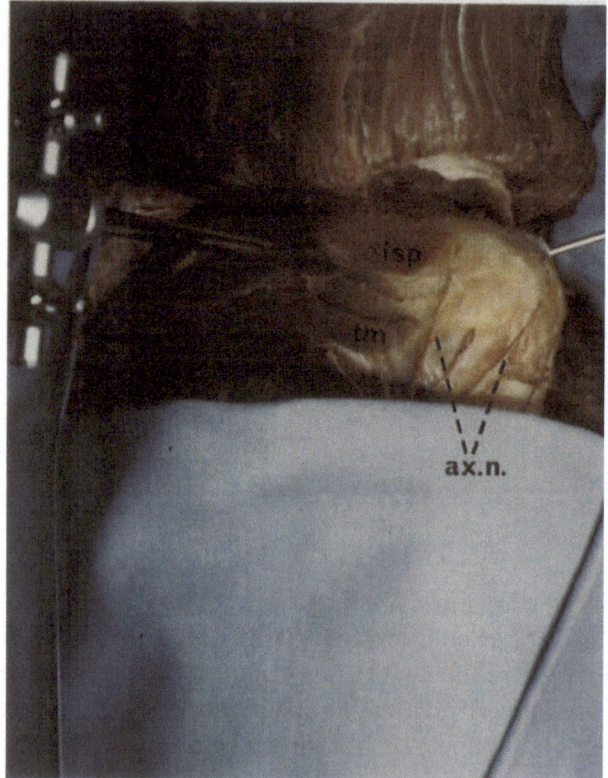

Fig. 32. Anatomical specimen. Correct positioning of arthroscope in the inferior portion of infraspinatus m. *ax.n.* Branches of axillary nerve dissected from deltoid m., *tm* teres minor m., *isp* infraspinatus m.

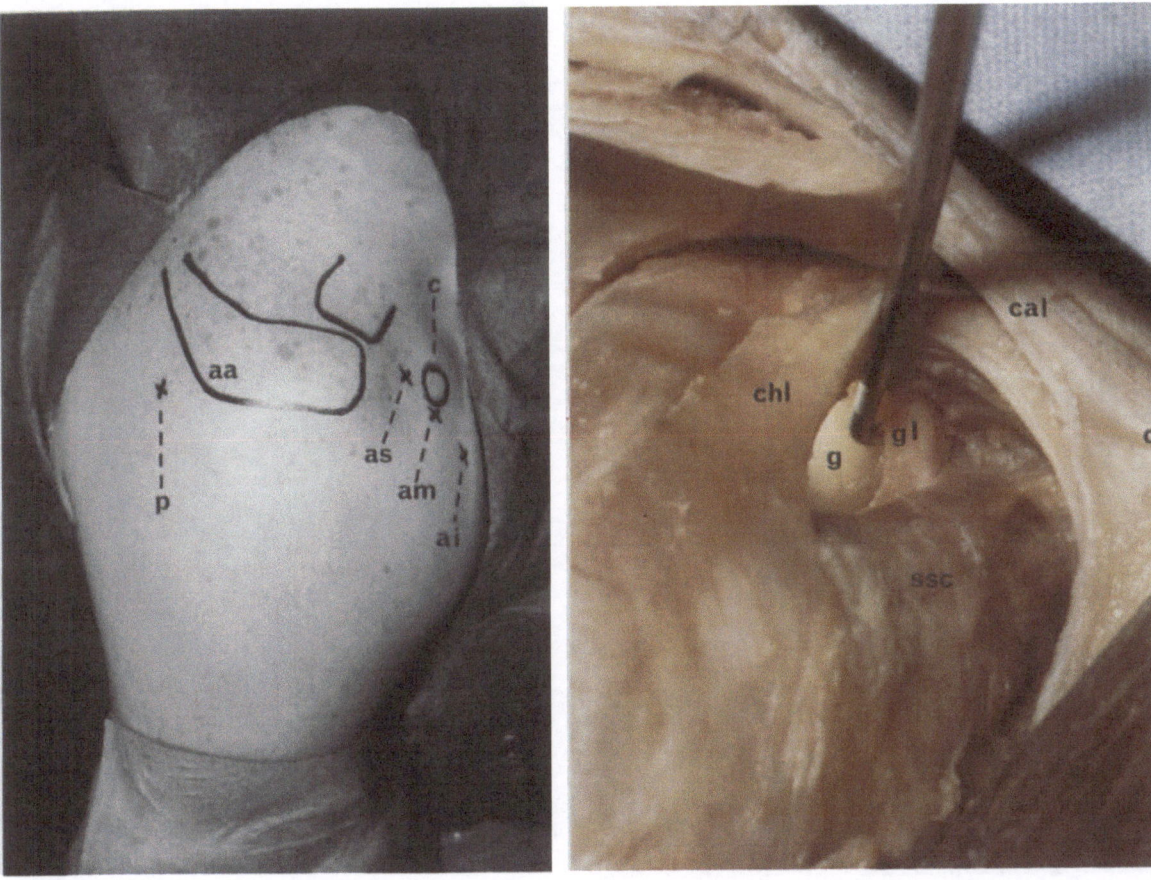

Fig. 33   Fig. 34

Fig. 33. Portals to glenohumeral joint. *p* Posterior portal, *as* antero-superior portal, *am* anterior middle portal, *ai* antero-inferior portal, *aa* acromial angle, *c* coracoid tip. Lateral view, patient in beach-chair position

Fig. 34. Anatomical specimen. Probe inserted into joint through standard portal, coracohumeral ligament displaced slightly cranially for better view. *g* Glenoid surface, *gl* glenoid labrum, *ssc* subscapularis m., *chl* coracohumeral ligament, *cal* coracoacromial ligament, *c* coracoid tip

Skin preparation and draping

Preparation for shoulder arthroscopy can be technically more demanding and time-consuming than for other joints. After threefold disinfection of the operative area, it is draped step by step. We use sterile self adhesive, waterproof hip drapes (Johnson & Johnson). It is important to keep the patient from getting wet and protect the patient from the sometimes considerable amount of cold irrigation fluid. The first self-adhesive drape is applied from below and placed in a way that the loose ends overlap in the lateral region of the neck. Subsequently, the arm and the elbow brace are wrapped in a sterile thigh stocking (Stockinette large, Mölnlycke). A longitudinal cut must be made in the stocking because of the

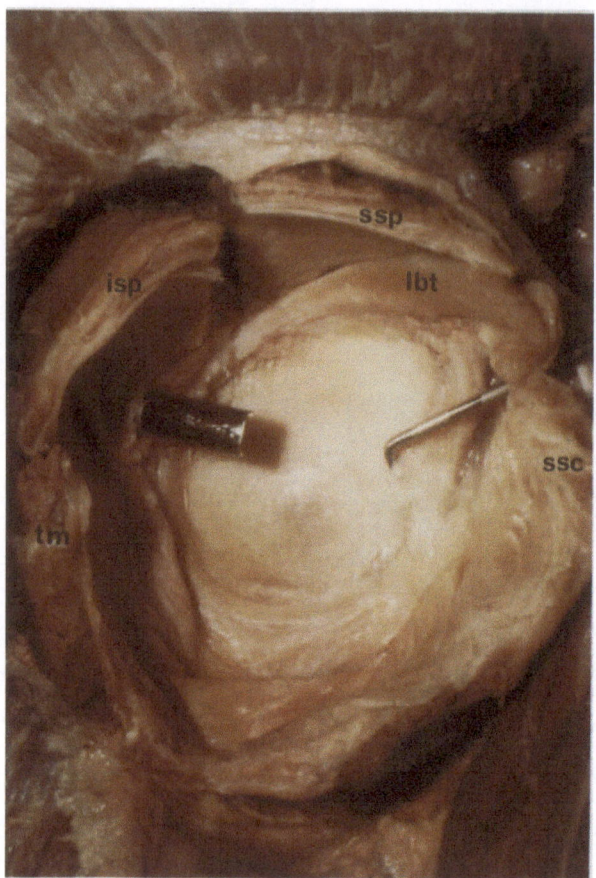

Fig. 35. Anatomical specimen. Shoulder joint socket with surrounding soft tissue, humeral head disarticulated. Arthroscope through posterior portal. Probe inserted through anterior middle portal. *ssc* Subscapularis tendon, *lbt* long biceps tendon, *ssp* supraspinatus tendon, *isp* infraspinatus tendon, *tm* teres minor m.

traction rope and it is subsequently fixed with adhesive tape and two small adhesive drapes so as to permit total sterile mobility of the arm. The second orthopedic hip drape is applied from above and it is positioned so as to effectively isolate the anesthetist from the surgical field. Draping is performed in the same way for both the lateral recumbent and "beach-chair" positions (Figs. 25 and 26).

Instrumentation

We use a standard set of instruments for diagnostic arthroscopy and bursoscopy and two special sets of instruments for therapeutic arthroscopic interventions in the glenohumeral joint and subacromial space.

Standard instrumentation (Fig. 27)

- Arthroscope. It consists of a 5 mm arthroscopic sheath with a blunt trocar and 30 and 70° wide-angle scopes. Normally the 30° scope is sufficient. For visualization of the

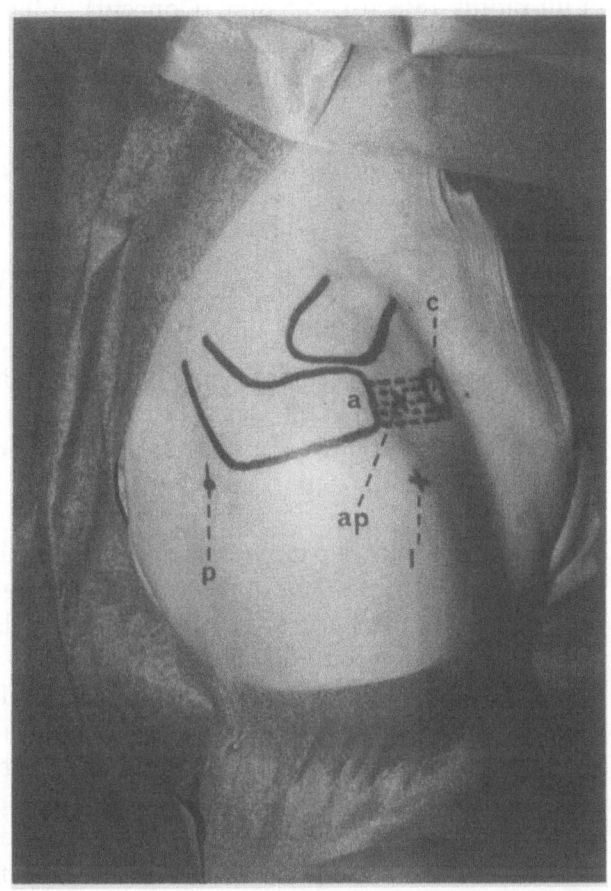

Fig. 36. Portal to subacromial space. Lateral view, patient in beach-chair position. *p* Posterior portal (scope), *l* lateral portal, *ap* anterior portal, *a* tip of acromion, *c* coracoid tip

subscapularis bursa and the evaluation of the posterior limbus from the standard posterior portal for the scope, however, the 70° scope is very useful. Therefore it should always be available as a reserve instrument.

- Probe. Palpation of the joint and subacromial space is imperative. In particular, detachments of the labrum can often not be diagnosed by inspection alone. It is only after manipulation with the probe that the lesion becomes visible. This is particularly the case with a S.L.A.P. lesion, which is often not detected until the biceps tendon is tensed with the probe. To palpate the rotator cuff, it may be necessary to use a curved probe, as the tendon close to its insertion is otherwise difficult to reach.
- Rongeur. This universal arthroscopic instrument is well suited to smooth cartilage and to debride tissue at the limbus and the rotator cuff.
- "Pit bull" (Acufex). These are sharp-pointed grasping forceps with a locking mechanism, used for the removal of loose bodies or larger resected portions of the labrum.
- Cushing cannula. A blunt cannula which can be inserted in case of poor vision to increase the outflow of the irrigation fluid.

- Full-radius resector, 5.5 mm (Concept). When performing bursoscopy, the use of a shaver may become necessary. Weblike bursal tissue must often be removed to ensure good vision in the subdeltoid bursa.

Instrumentation for procedures in the glenohumeral joint
(arthroscopic Bankart screw fixation technique, arthroscopic Bankart suture repair)
(Fig. 28)

These special operative techniques require several supplementary instruments. A detailed description of the individual operative techniques is given in Chaps. 6.1 and 6.3.

- Shoulder elevator (Acufex). This thin rasplike instrument is used to mobilize the labrum and the periosteum at the glenoid rim in recurrent or habitual dislocation of the shoulder.
- Bankart rasp (Acufex). In contrast to the shoulder elevator, the undersurface of the Bankart rasp is like a coarse file. It is used to freshen-up the glenoid rim beneath the labral lesion.
- Arthroplasty burr, 4.5 mm (Concept). When performing an arthroscopic Bankart operation, a bony groove should be created at the glenoid rim with the ball-headed burr. As the ball tip of the burr is very sharp, the cartilage may be damaged if the instrument is operated in the wrong direction of rotation.
- Resch labrum screw fixation set (Leibinger). This set consists of a serrated trocar sheath with a handle into which a trocar with a conical tip and a 1 mm central canal is inserted. With a 1 mm guide wire the capsule and labrum are picked up and the pin is placed 3–4 mm from the glenoid rim. The cannulated titanium screws and shims are inserted over the guide wire. This instrumentation is used for extraarticular limbus screw fixation in the case of recurrent shoulder dislocation, intraarticular screw fixation of a S.L.A.P. lesion as well as extra- or intraarticular screw fixation of a bony glenoid rim avulsion (Chap. 6.3).
- Glötzer limbus suture set. This consists of a cannula with two communicating lumina, through which two Bankart pins are drilled through the glenoid rim. Absorbable suture material is threaded through the eyes of the pins. They are then pulled through posteriorly and the suture tails are tied subcutaneously. This method corresponds with a modified Kessler suture (see Chap. 6.1).

Instrumentation for arthroscopic subacromial decompression (Fig. 29)

For arthroscopic acromioplasty we use a supplementary standardized set of instruments. For detailed information on the technique see Chap. 7.1.

- Sterile marker pencil. Delineation of the important landmarks greatly facilitates orientation, especially following swelling of the shoulder.
- Full-radius resector 5.5 mm (Concept). This shaver attachment is the most suitable for removal of soft tissue from the undersurface of the acromion.
- Hypodermic needles. Conventional injection needles are used for percutaneous delineation of the important anatomical structures.

- Resch ligament forceps and sliding knife (Leibinger). These two instruments are used to simultaneously dissect and resect the coracoacromial ligament. The peculiarity of these grasping forceps with a locking mechanism is that the jaws are of different lengths, which allows introduction and advancement of the shorter upper jaw along the upper surface of the ligament. The sliding knife has a U-shaped profile in cross-section, the sharp tip is bevelled. It is advanced over the ligament forceps so that the ligament is simultaneously dissected and partially resected by the two lateral blades. (These instruments are rarely used now that we have changed our standard procedure, see Chap. 7.)
- Electrosurgical knife. This is used for cautery and coagulation of the soft tissues on the undersurface of the acromion, thereby facilitating their removal.
- Reciprocating file (reciprocating saw, Hall/Zimmer). We use this compressed air operated file for removal of the cancellous bone from the undersurface of the acromion as an alternative to the "acromionizer". Osteophytes on the undersurface of the lateral clavicle can also be removed with this instrument. A variety of different files are available, thus allowing accurate control of the extent of the bony resection (Chap. 7).
- Tapered or oval burr, 6 mm "Acromionizer" (Concept). This is a shaver attachment specially designed for acromioplasty with a 1 cm oval burr (Fig. 30).

Portals

To standardize the portals for arthroscopic interventions in the shoulder joint, it is useful to delineate the important anatomical landmarks with a sterile colored pencil before the operation.

These landmarks are:

- the acromion,
- the lateral clavicle,
- the acromio-clavicular joint,
- the coracoid tip.

Using these landmarks as references, the points of incision for the different portals are marked with crosses. The portals for the glenohumeral joint and the subacromial space are described below.

Portals to the glenohumeral joint

- Posterior portal (for the arthroscope). This is the standard portal for the scope. Usually the joint is punctured at the start of the operation. The site of entry is 1 cm inferior and 1.5 cm medial to the acromial angle; the needle is advanced towards the coracoid tip. After perforating the joint, it is distended with Ringer's lactate. Correct intraarticular location of the needle is confirmed by the return of the clear injection fluid after the removal of the syringe. Distending the joint facilitates the introduction of the trocar. However, it is not absolutely necessary if the surgeon is sufficiently experienced.
  The skin incision is also made 1.5 cm medial and 1 cm inferior to the acromial angle of the scapula. Normally, the incision would be made 2 cm inferior to it, but this usually makes

access to the subacromial space from the same incision more difficult. Locating the portal slightly higher has no disadvantages whatsoever for arthroscopy of the glenohumeral joint. The incision is only down to the subcutaneous layer. Subsequently, the arthroscopic sheath with the blunt trocar is inserted and carefully advanced towards the humeral head. The surgeon's other hand grasps the head of the humerus in such a way that translation of the head can be felt with the fingertips when the trocar reaches the humeral head (Fig. 31). The trocar is then passed medially until the gap between the humeral head and the glenoid rim is found. The assistant surgeon distracts the humeral head from the socket as far as possible by grasping the proximal shaft of the humerus. This manoeuvre makes room for the insertion of the trocar and simultaneously tenses the capsule. The sheath of the scope is now turned towards the coracoid tip in a medial direction in order to reach the triangle between head, socket and rotator cuff. Only then is the capsule perforated. The sheath must be advanced with care.

The correct site of insertion is located in the superior one-third of the capsule, in the triangle described above (socket−head−rotatur cuff) and passes through the infraspinatus muscle. Anatomical dissection shows that the instrument should not damage any important vessels or nerves in this position (Fig. 32).

● Anterior portal (for instrumentation) [6, 8, 10]. We distinguish between 3 anterior portals in the glenohumeral joint:
− anterior middle portal (standard portal),
− antero-superior portal,
− antero-inferior portal (Fig. 33).

Standard portal.   The skin incision is made slightly lateral to and at the level of the coracoid tip. The scalpel should only cut the skin in order to avoid perforating branches of the cephalic vein. The incision should be as small as possible as only the probe is used initially. It is advanced through the muscles until it reaches the anterior capsule, between the upper margin of the subscapularis tendon and the coracohumeral ligament (Figs. 34 and 35). Before perforating the capsule, the scope is advanced to the anterior glenoid rim to check the correct insertion of the instrument into the joint. The capsule is perforated with rotatory movements. The following procedures in the glenohumeral joint can be carried out via this portal:

− diagnostic arthroscopy,
− resection and shaving of the labrum,
− removal of loose bodies in the joint,
− limbus reattachment in the antero-superior and middle portion of the glenoid rim.

Although the antero-inferior portion of the limbus can be reached through this portal by displacing the subscapularis tendon in an inferior direction, limbus fixation with screw or suture is not possible.

A Wissinger rod may be useful for accurate placement of the standard portal. After having brought the scope close to the upper margin of the subscapularis tendon, it is replaced in the sheath by the Wissinger rod, which is then advanced to just below the skin. A skin incision is made where it bulges out and the 4 mm guiding trocar and the 7 mm universal cannula are inserted with rotatory movements into the joint over the Wissinger rot. Finally, the rod is again replaced by the scope.

Antero-inferior portal.   An incision is made 1.5–2 cm inferior and slightly lateral to the coracoid tip. This portal passes through the substance of the subscapular muscle. We use this portal in cases for arthroscopic extraarticular Bankart fixation technique and extraarticular Bankart suture repair (see Chaps. 6.1 and 6.3).

Antero-superior portal.   A skin incision is made 1 cm superior to the coracoid tip. The joint is entered slightly anterior to the long biceps tendon. This portal is used as an additional portal for instrumentation when performing arthroscopic operations at the anterior glenoid rim (e.g., additional insertion of the probe to reduce a fragment of the glenoid rim in the course of an arthroscopic screw fixation; the distance between the instruments, which are inserted anteriorly at the same time, is increased) (Chap. 6.3).

If a more detailed evaluation of the anterior glenoid rim with visualization of the inferior recesses at the scapular neck becomes necessary, the scope is introduced from an anterior direction through a universal cannula. The antero-superior portal is ideally suited also for this purpose.

Portals to the subacromial space (bursoscopy) (Fig. 36)

- Posterior portal (for the arthroscope). This portal corresponds with the portal for the scope at arthroscopy as a bursoscopy is never performed without first inspecting the glenohumeral joint. After having replaced the arthroscope with the blunt trocar, the sheath is angled slightly inferiorly and slowly withdrawn. When withdrawing from the rotator cuff, a slight snapping can be felt. Subsequently, the sheath is advanced under the acromion. (Attention: Previous distension of the subdeltoid bursa using a mixture of 18 ml saline solution and 2 ml vasopressin (POR 8) facilitates insertion of the instruments).
- Lateral portal (for instrumentation). The skin incision is made approx. 2 cm lateral to the anterior end of the acromion. The following instruments for bursoscopic procedures are inserted through this portal:

- probe,
- shaver,
- ligament grasping forceps with sliding knife,
- rongeur,
- electrosurgical knife,
- acromionizer.

If no universal cannula is used, the instruments must be inserted very carefully, as repeated changes may severely damage the deltoid muscle.
- Anterior portal (reciprocating file). The skin incision is made 1 cm anterior to the mid-point of the anterior end of the acromion. The incision is usually located in the same sagittal plane as the posterior portal and this may be useful for orientation. The recipro-cating file is inserted through this portal, so the skin incision should just allow passage of the head of the file. If the incision is too big, a large volume of irrigation fluid will

escape when using the file, and this can severely impair vision (pressure decrease in the subacromial space) (see Chap. 7).

References

1. Andrews JR, Carson WG, Ortega K (1984) Arthroscopy of the shoulder: technique and normal anatomy. Am J Sports Med 12:1–7
2. Blachut PA, Day B (1989) Arthroscopic anatomy of the shoulder. Arthrosc Related Surg 5:1–10
3. Cofield RH (1983) Arthroscopy of the shoulder. Mayo Clin Proc 58:501–508
4. Johnson LL (1980) Arthroscopy of the shoulder. Orthop Clin N Amer 11:197–204
5. Johnson LL (1987) The shoulder joint. An arthroscopist's perspective of anatomy and pathology. Clin Orthop 223:113–125
6. Matthews LS, Terry G, Vetter WL (1985) Shoulder anatomy for the arthroscopist. Arthroscopy 1:83–91
7. Ogilvie-Harris DJ, Wiley AM (1986) Arthroscopic surgery of the shoulder. A general appraisal. J Bone Joint Surg [Br] 68:201–207
8. Seiler H (1990) Diagnostische Arthroskopie. In: Habermeyer P (ed) Schulterchirurgie. Urban & Schwarzenberg, München, pp 128–135
9. Skyhar MJ, Altchek DW, Warren RF, Wickiewicz TL, O'Brien SJ (1988) Shoulder arthroscopy with the patient in the beach-chair position. Arthroscopy 4:256–259
10. Wolf EM (1989) Anterior portals in shoulder arthroscopy. Arthroscopy 5:201–208

4 Diagnostic arthroscopy

H. Thöni, H. Resch, and G. Sperner

The anatomical structure of the shoulder joint is eminently suited to arthroscopic examination. The joint itself is spacious, the capsule is loose; according to Fick a second humeral head would fit into the joint [10, 25]. From an anatomical point of view the placement of arthroscopic portals may be somewhat more difficult than in the knee joint, but they are equally nontraumatic and safe, provided a few clear rules are followed [6].

Advances in open surgery of the shoulder joint, combined with increasing accuracy and innovations in diagnostic techniques (CT, MRI, sonography) produced a new understanding of the joint but also raised new questions. These have been more readily answered with arthroscopic techniques, with the ability to assimilate anatomical and functional parameters proving particularly useful. An added benefit of arthroscopy was a reduction in morbidity and rehabilitation time following surgical intervention [8].

Arthroscopy has proven to be an invaluable diagnostic technique as well as an excellent means of procedural surgery in the shoulder joint, given appropriate indications.

Indications

In the assessment of injuries and diseases in the shoulder joint there are a number of methods of examination, including arthroscopy, a relatively invasive and time-consuming method, which should be the last step in establishing a diagnosis [5].

Standard history taking, physical examination and radiology usually provide a tentative diagnosis and suggest further steps in the assessment. Special radiological views can supply detailed pictures of fractures and of secondary changes to the bony skeleton, whereas sonography is used to examine the rotator cuff and the biceps tendon. More precise localization of fractures, especially of the scapula, and the extent of arthritic changes can be determined by plain computed tomography. In the case of instability, double-contrast computed tomography may be used to choose the adequate surgical method and to determine whether or not arthroscopic repair is appropriate.

Arthrography may identify lesions of the rotator cuff which went undetected during sonography, such as small or incomplete tears on the synovial aspect, and may confirm the diagnosis of a frozen shoulder.

Nuclear magnetic resonance imaging readily visualizes the muscles and tendons of the shoulder joint. Since it is an expensive and time-consuming examination, this method is not yet used routinely.

If any important questions remain unresolved, diagnostic arthroscopy is indicated, however, as clinical experience and diagnostic accuracy increase, it is used more and more for the confirmation and grading of the diagnosis. Then, if corresponding findings are established, and technical qualification and equipment are appropriate, arthroscopic surgery may be subsequently performed.

Indications for arthroscopy of the shoulder joint:

- anterior subluxation,
- traumatic initial dislocation,
- multidirectional instability,
- unclear direction of a dislocation,
- loose bodies in the joint,
- frozen shoulder,
- infection of the joint,
- impingement syndrome,
- unspecific pain, refractory to treatment.

Recurrent anterior subluxation.   The patient complains of sudden sharp pains (dead arm syndrome) and a feeling of instability when the abducted arm is externally rotated (tennis serve). Physical examination shows a negative impingement test, but a highly positive apprehension test [20].

Traumatic initial dislocation.   If a patient who engages in sports such as rock-climbing or white-water canoeing has an acute dislocation of the shoulder, he could be in serious danger should the dislocation re-occur. In such circumstances, arthroscopic evaluation of the damage and its repair are recommended [16, 25].

Multidirectional instability.   The arthroscopic detection of secondary lesions of the head or socket may improve the prognosis of a possible surgical intervention.

Unclear direction of dislocation.   If the direction of a recurrent or habitual dislocation of the shoulder cannot be determined using computed tomography, arthroscopy with simultaneous functional dynamic examination may be helpful in clarifying the situation [11].

Suspected loose bodies in the joint.   Recurrent locking or intraarticular snapping or clicking, possibly with positive radiographic findings, are indications for arthroscopy, which then provides information regarding the site of origin and genesis; arthroscopic removal is usually accomplished without difficulty.

Frozen shoulder.   An idiopathic adhesive capsulitis can be mobilized carefully by means of a so-called distension arthroscopy with forced filling of the joint [21].

Infected shoulder joint.   The shoulder joint is irrigated arthroscopically and the extent of the infection determined [11]. If necessary, it is possible to perform partial synovectomy using a shaver and to place a suction-irrigation drain.

Impingement syndrome.   If the rotator cuff is sonographically and arthrographically intact and the LA-test positive, and the patient has failed to respond to conservative treatment after 6 months, acromioplasty is indicated. Prior to this intervention a so-called secondary impingement with damage to the limbus at the antero-superior rim of the socket should be excluded by means of arthroscopy (see Chap. 6.3).

Nonspecific pain in the shoulder refractory to treatment.   This is one of the few indications for initially only performing diagnostic arthroscopy.

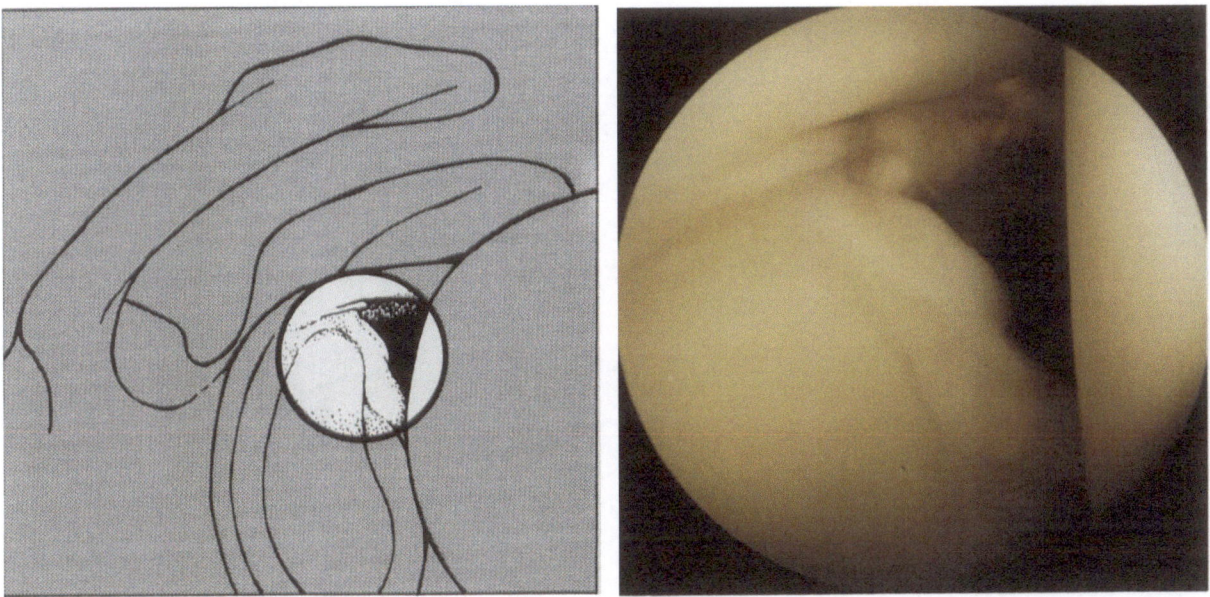

Fig. 37. Intact anterosuperior labrum: the origin of the long biceps tendon blends with the superiormost portion of the labrum

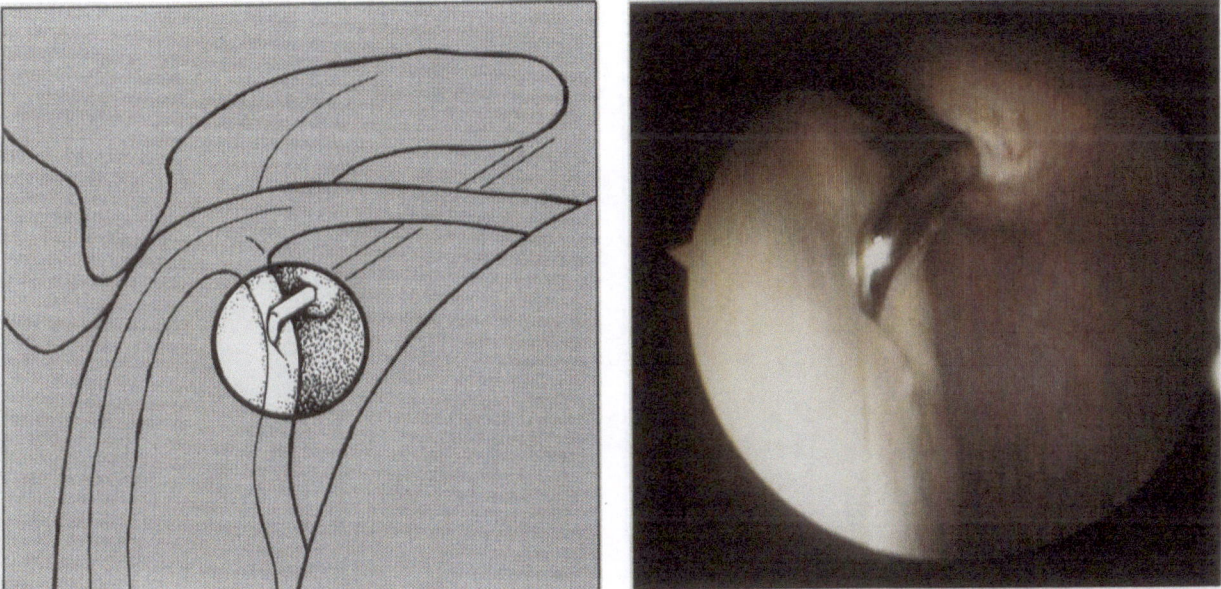

Fig. 38. Palpation of the anterior labrum to determine its firmness: it is noted to be intact. Note that the probe is inserted into the joint superior to the subscapularis tendon

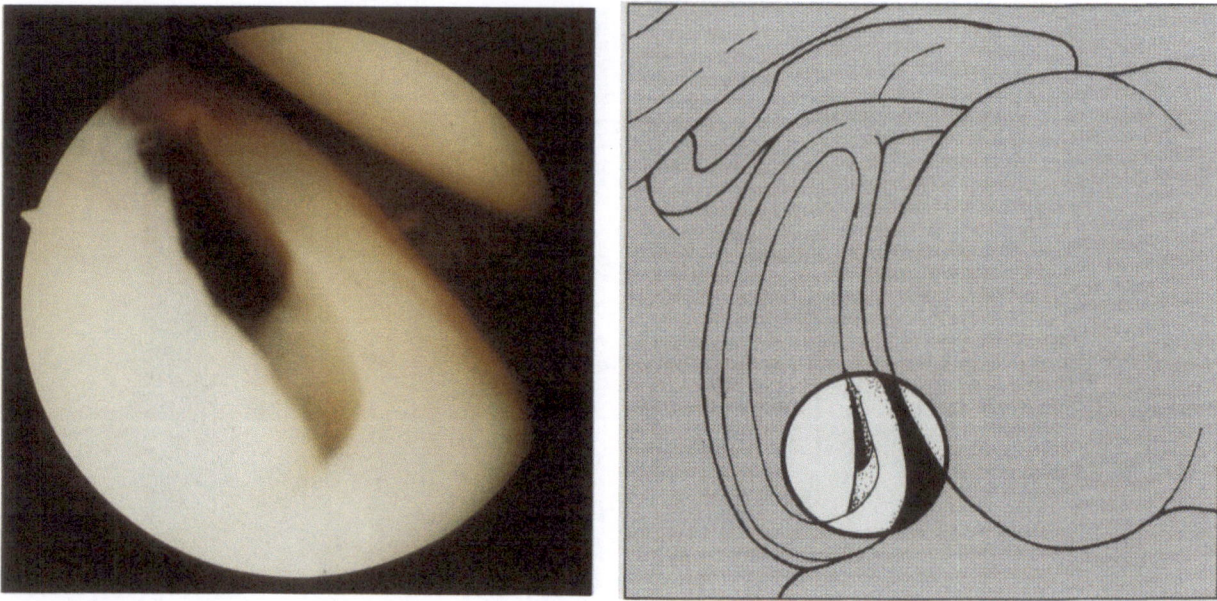

Fig. 39. Antero-inferior detachment of the glenoid labrum: Bankart lesion

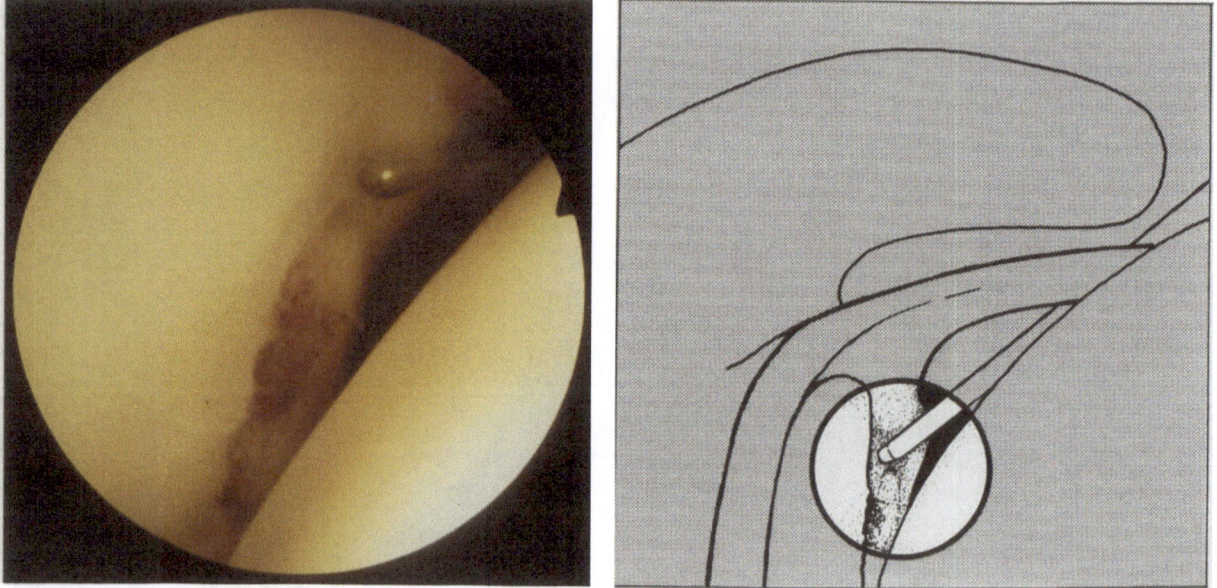

Fig. 40. Traumatic detachment of the anterior glenoid labrum in the region of the glenoid notch is noted to be recent due to adherent spots of bleeding

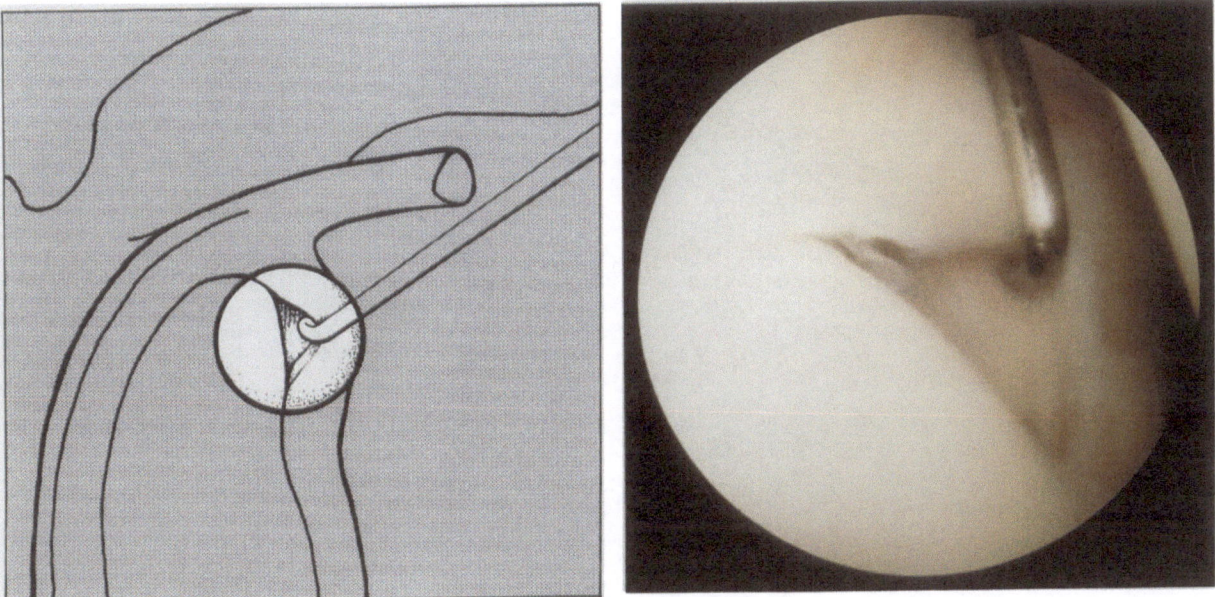

Fig. 41. Antero-superior detachment of the glenoid labrum at the rim of the socket: Andrews lesion

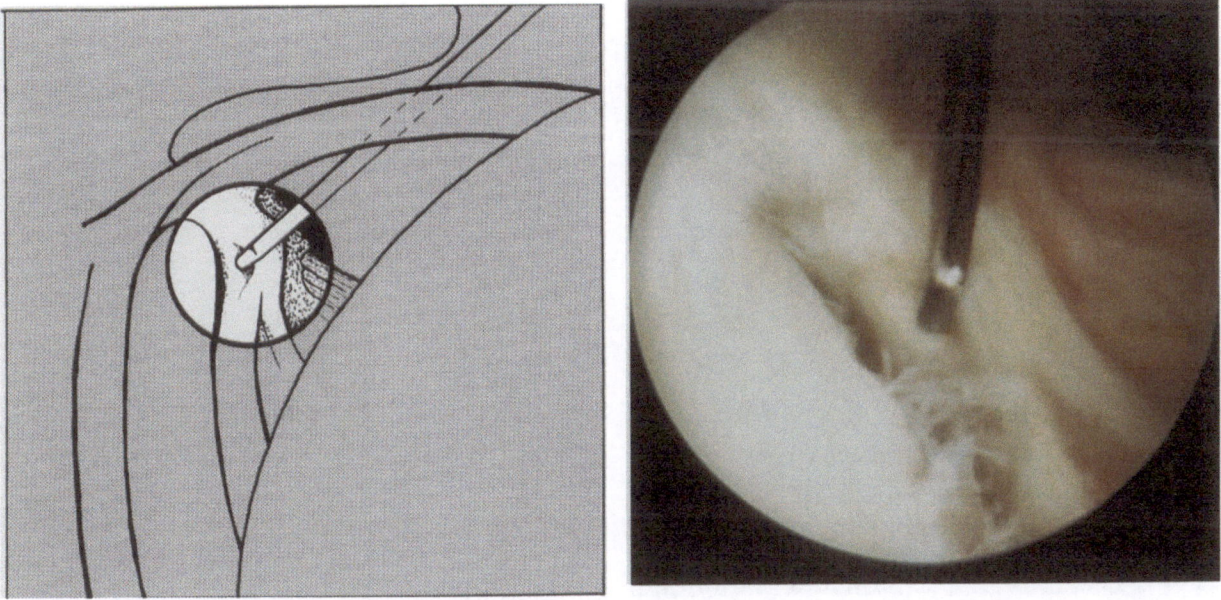

Fig. 42. Labral detachment at the antero-superior rim of the socket and associated insufficiency of the glenohumeral ligaments

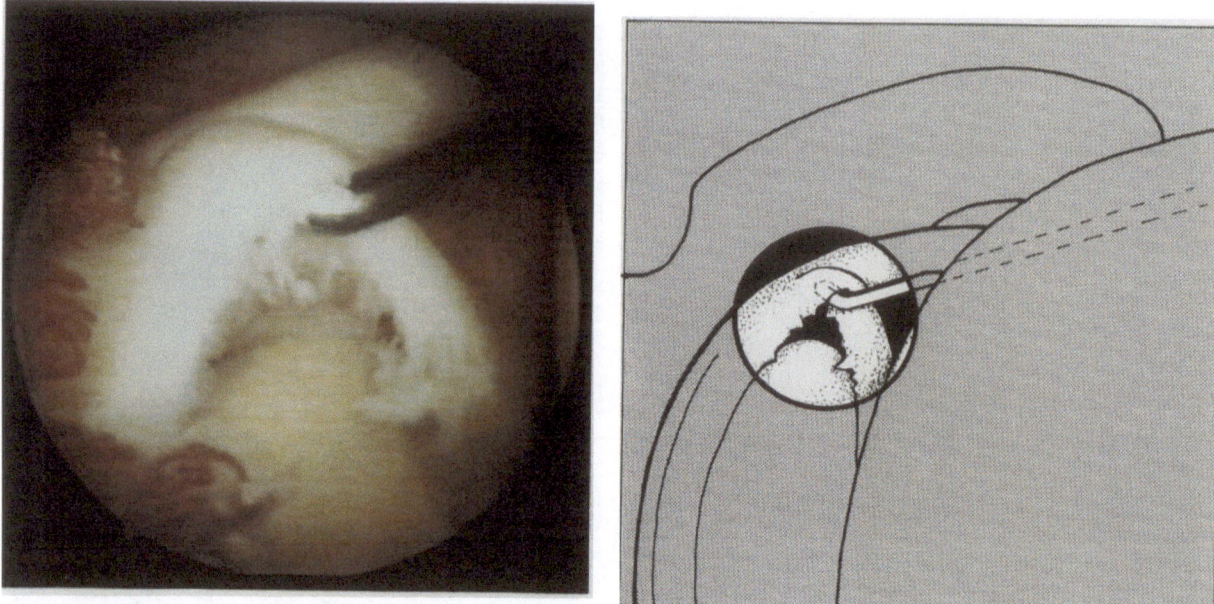

Fig. 43. Hood-like detachment of the glenoid labrum at the upper socket pole including the insertion of the biceps tendon: S.L.A.P. lesion. Synovitic changes in the surrounding area

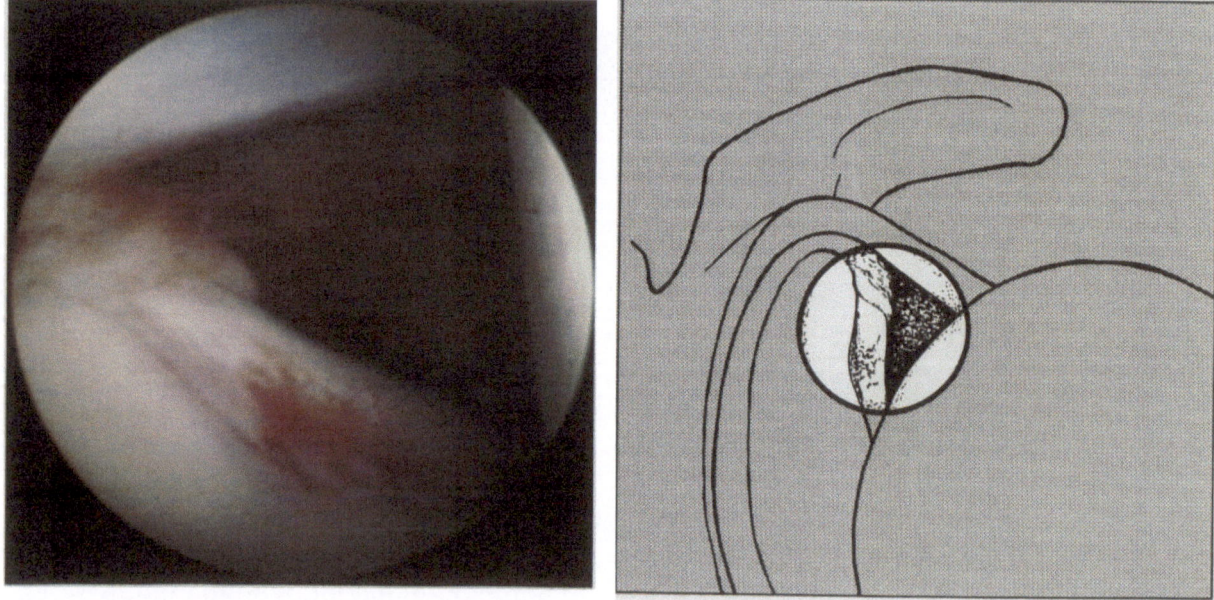

Fig. 44. Reddening as a sign of synovitis at the antero-superior labrum and the adjacent anterior wall of the shoulder: secondary impingement?

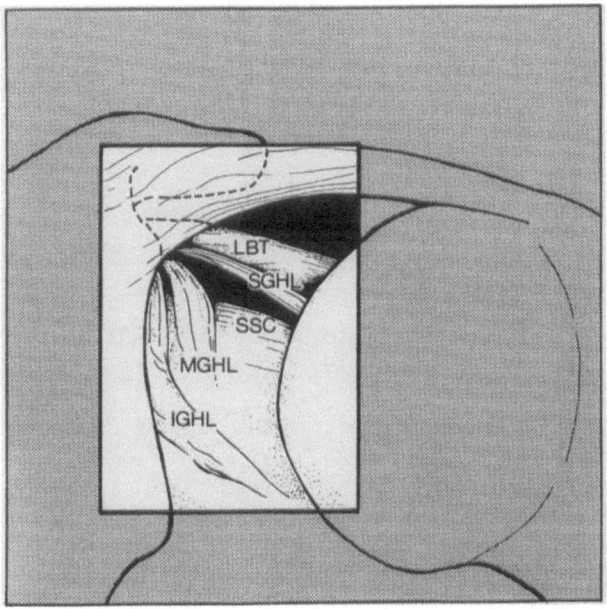

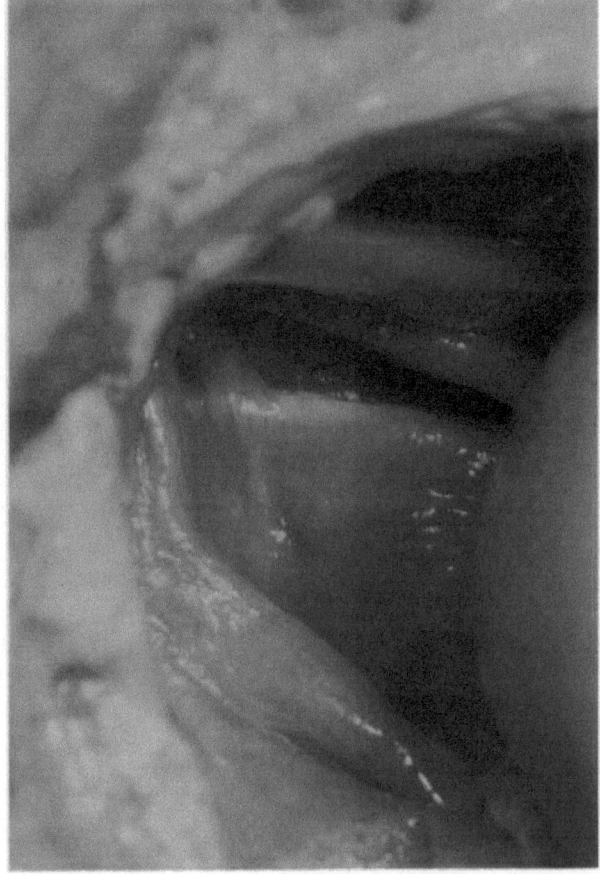

Fig. 45. Anatomical specimen of the anterior wall of the shoulder (intraarticular view from posterior, socket invisible because viewed tangentially). *LBT* Long biceps tendon, *SGHL* superior glenohumeral ligament, *SSC* subscapularis tendon, *MGHL* middle glenohumeral ligament, *IGHL* inferior glenohumeral ligament

Surgical technique

Anesthesia

Regional anesthesia by interscalene block has now probably become the method of choice when performing diagnostic arthroscopy of the shoulder. If intervention in the subacromial space becomes necessary or the patient does not want regional anesthesia, general anesthesia is required. The latter permits a reduction of bleeding through controlled hypotension; bleeding into the glenohumeral joint rarely causes problems with arthroscopy (Chap. 2).

Positioning

Lateral recumbent positioning of the patient with the upper part of the body in posterior inclination necessitates repositioning, renewed skin preparation and draping when changing to an open procedure. Only open acromioplasty can be carried out without changing the position of the patient [18].

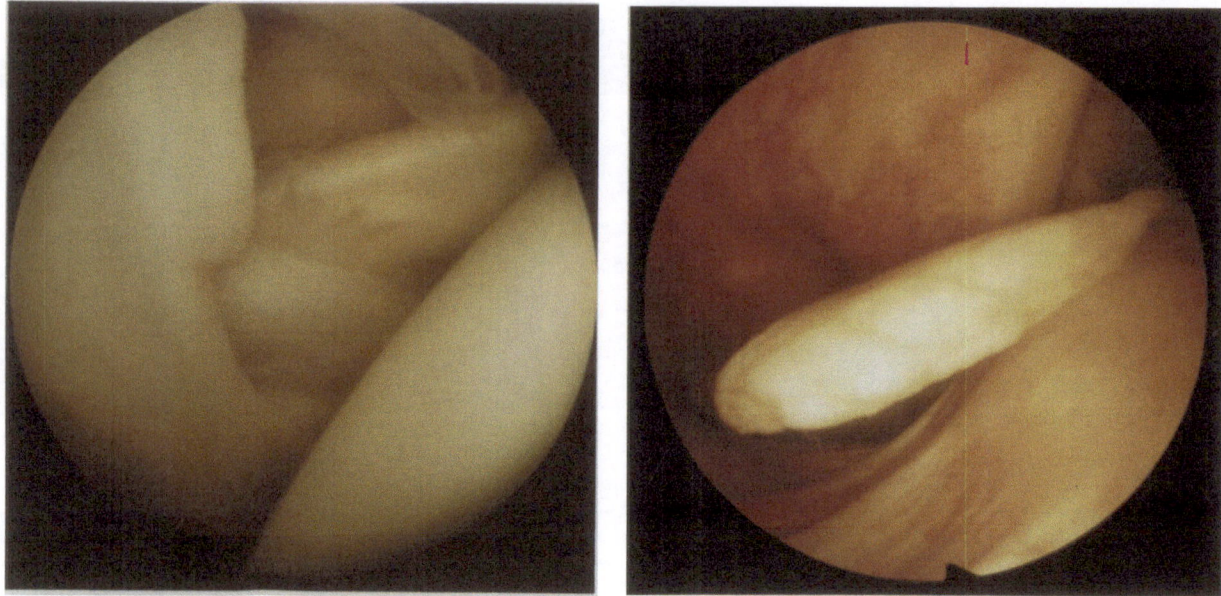

Fig. 46. Anterior shoulder wall of a healthy right shoulder: intact glenoid labrum; prominent upper margin of the subscapularis tendon; the middle glenohumeral ligament extending inferolaterally at an acute angle

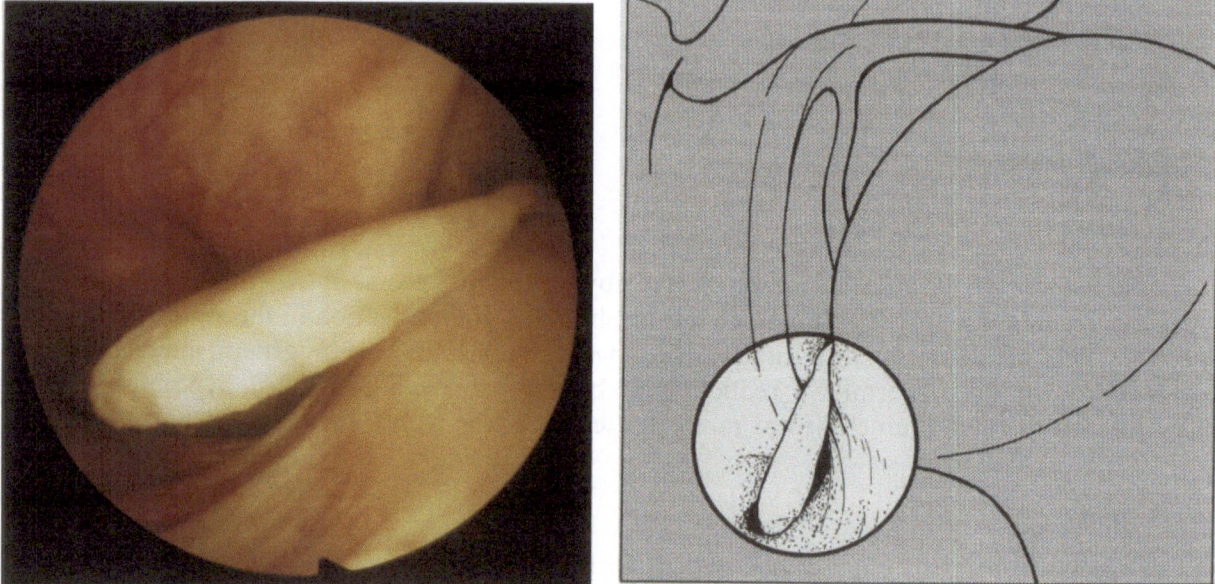

Fig. 47. Loose body in the axillary recess (site of predilection); the postero-inferior portion of the rim of the socket is visible

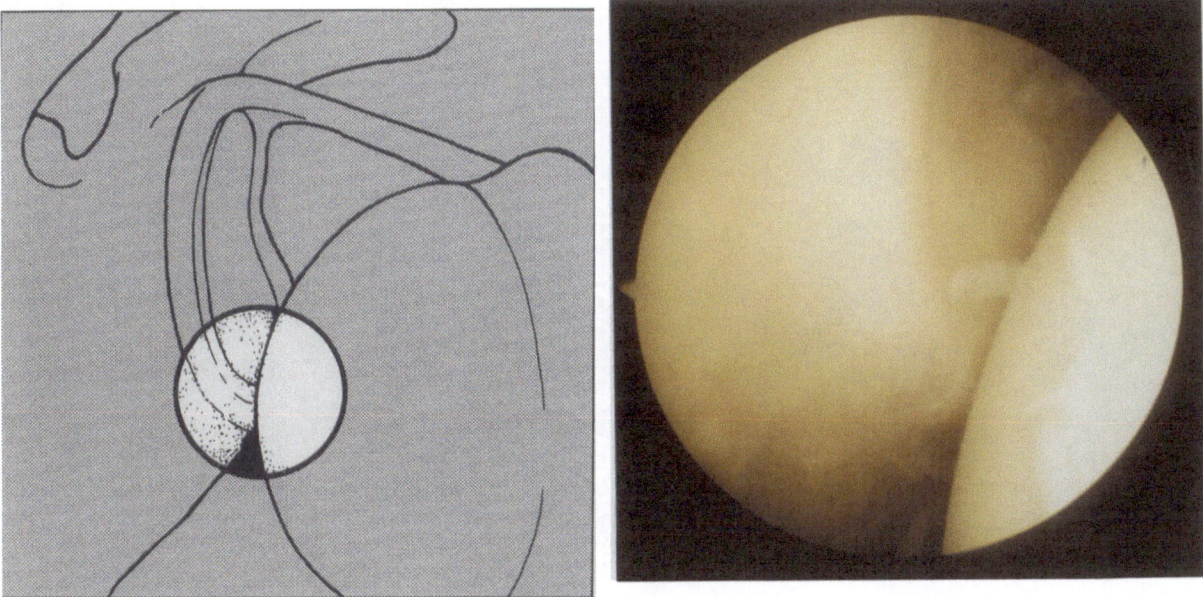

Fig. 48. Postero-inferior rim of the socket with intact flat glenoid labrum; central cartilage damage of the glenoid surface

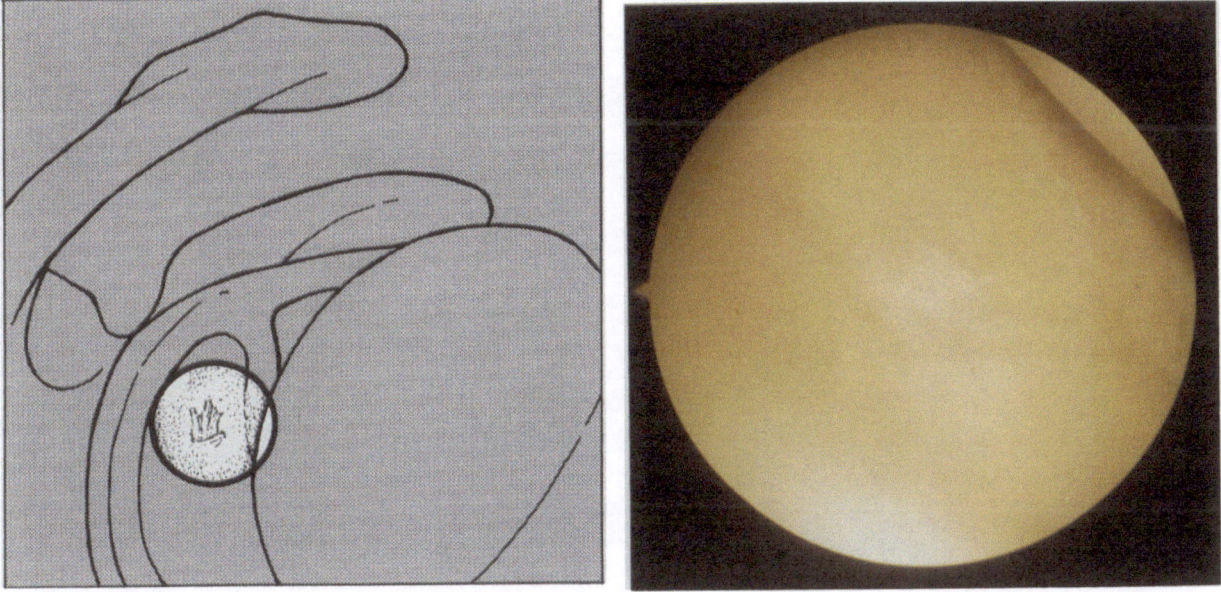

Fig. 49. Glenoid surface with central cartilage damage (the cartilage covering is thinnest at this point); the glenoid labrum visible at the notch is intact

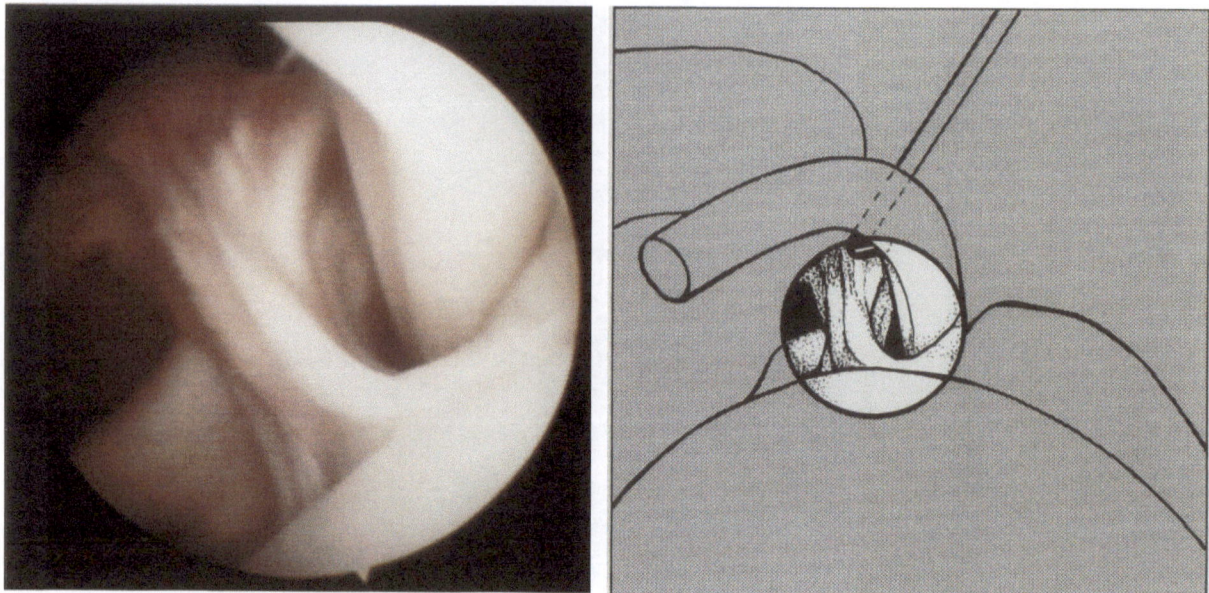

Fig. 50. Entrance of the biceps tendon into the intertubercular notch; surrounded by a branch of the superior glenohumeral ligament on the posterior side, medially the upper margin of the subscapularis tendon is still visible

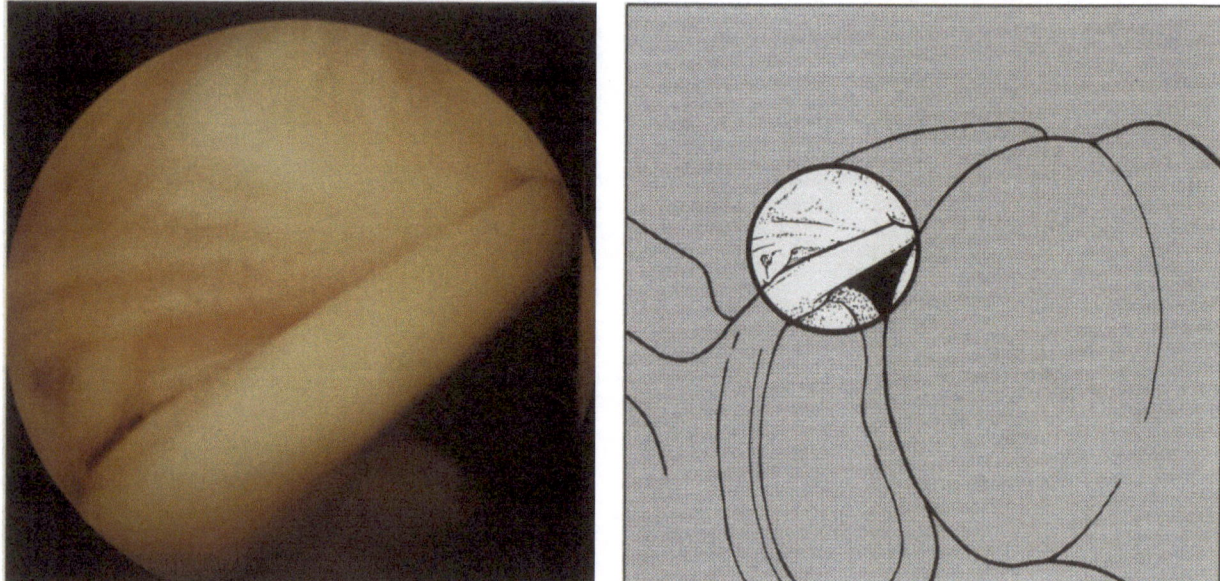

Fig. 51. Oblique course of the biceps tendon, extending from the superior pole of the socket over the humeral head in an antero-lateral direction; biceps tendon and visible portion of the rotator cuff are unremarkable

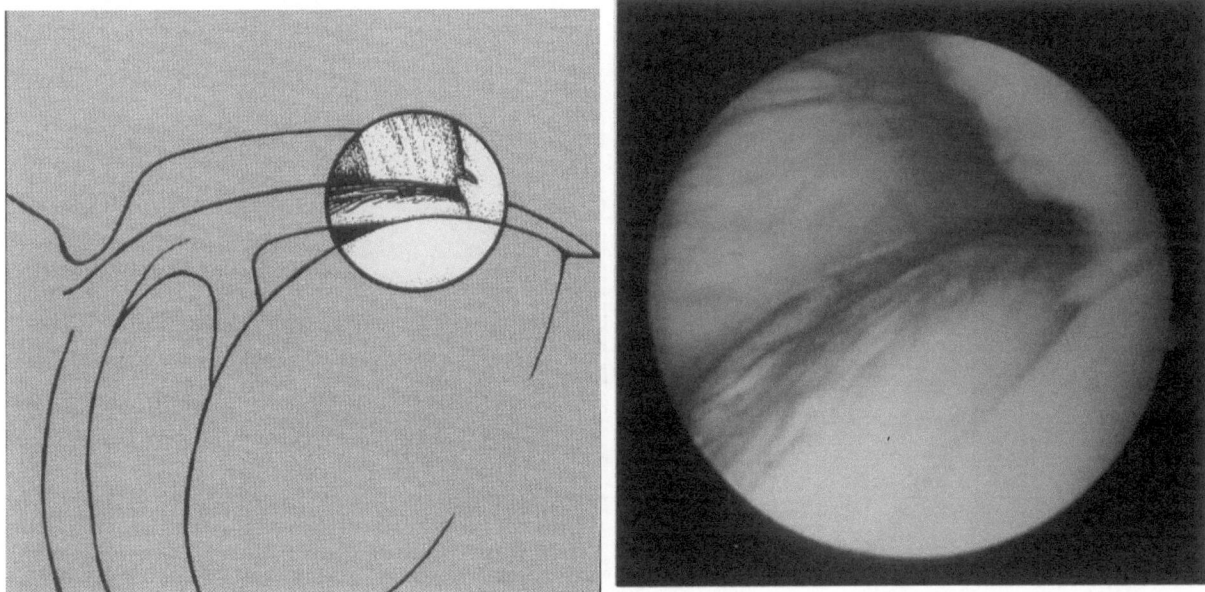

Fig. 52. Synovitis of the long biceps tendon at the entrance into the intertubercular notch, the adjacent rotator cuff is partially torn

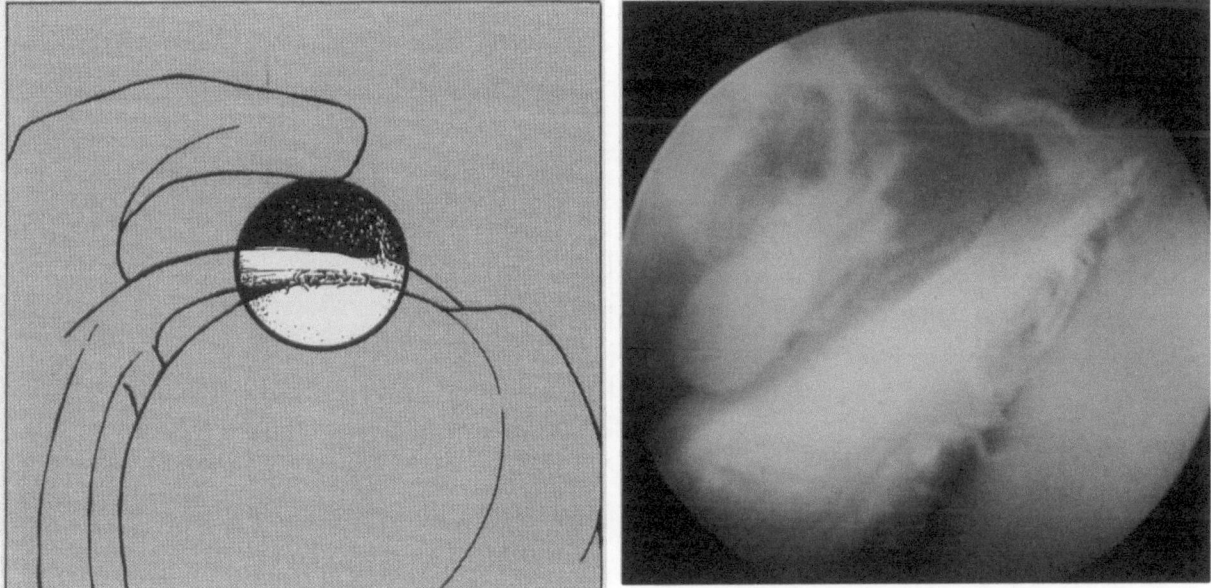

Fig. 53. Frayed, thinned biceps tendon; the adjacent rotator cuff is covered by synovitis pannus

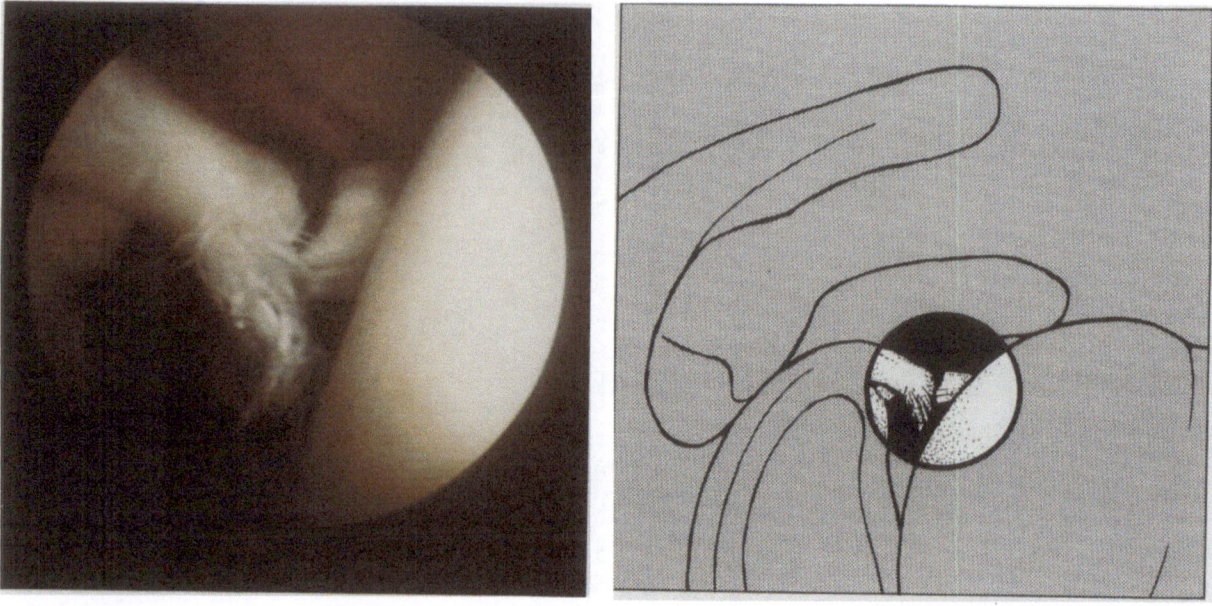

Fig. 54. Partial tear and degeneration of the long biceps tendon; in the background synovitis of the rotator cuff

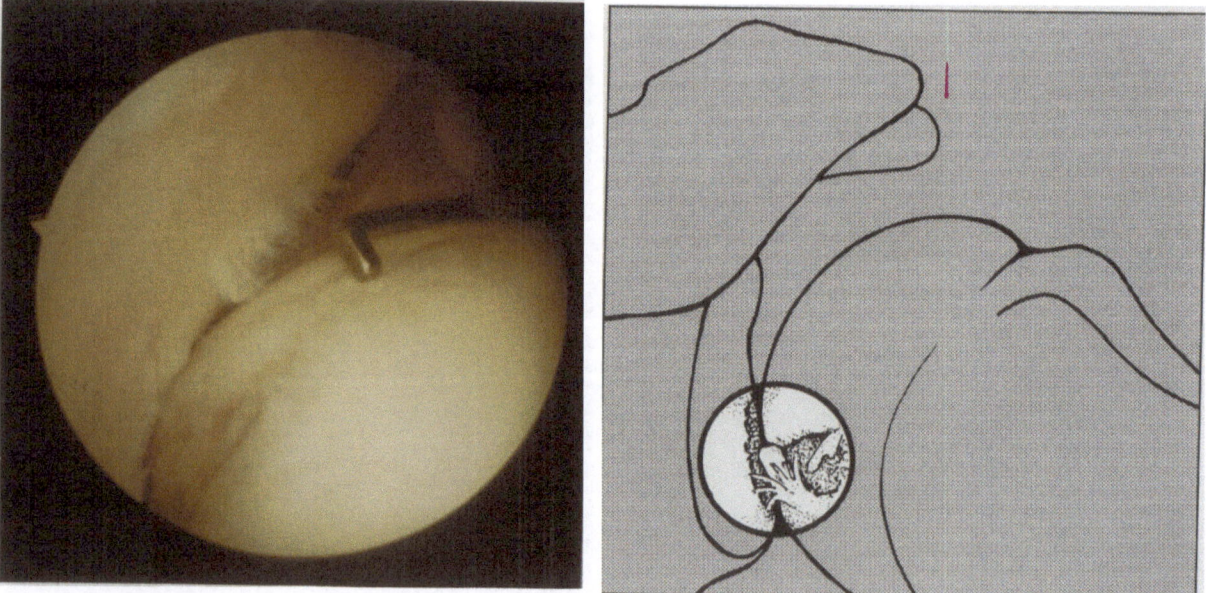

Fig. 55. Purely chondral damage to the humeral head due to recurrent subluxation, corresponding cartilage lesion at the anterior margin of the glenoid surface

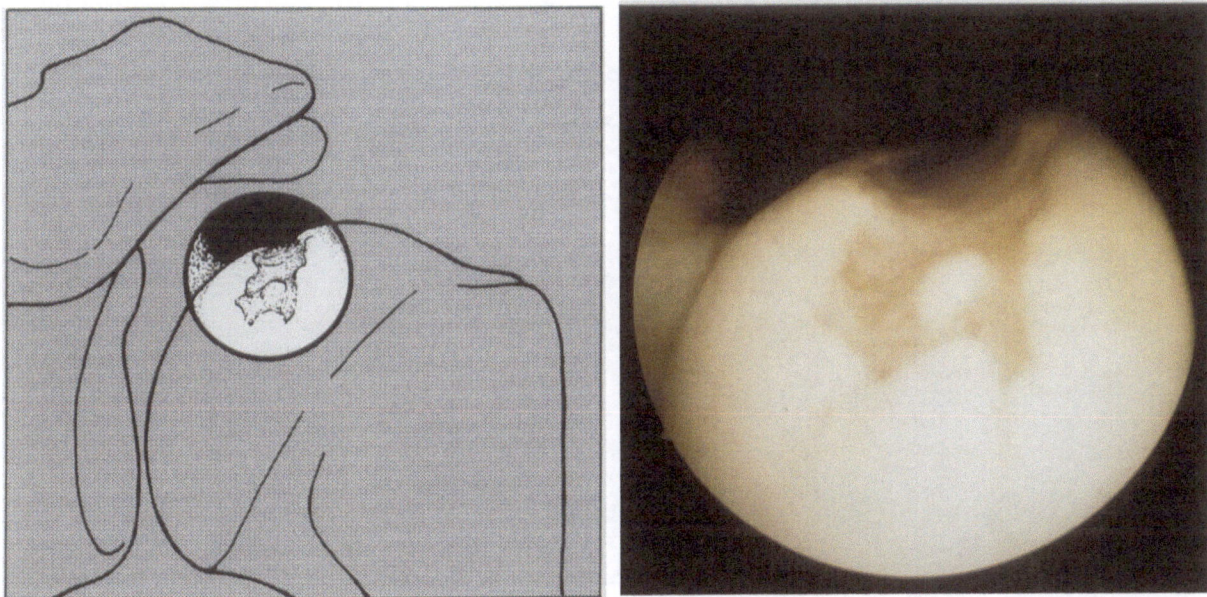

Fig. 56. Hill-Sachs lesion at the postero-lateral aspect of humeral head; the depressed osteochondral fracture is already rounded off and smoothed – it is old

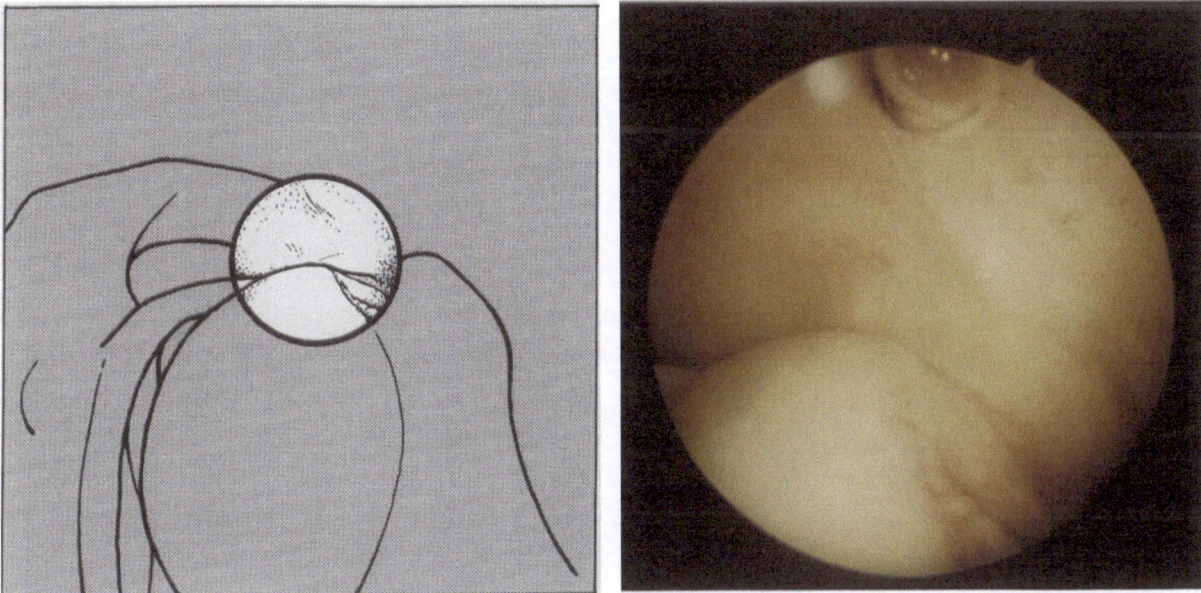

Fig. 57. Attachment of the rotator cuff at the edge of the cartilage covering the head (folds next to the redundant synovial fold)

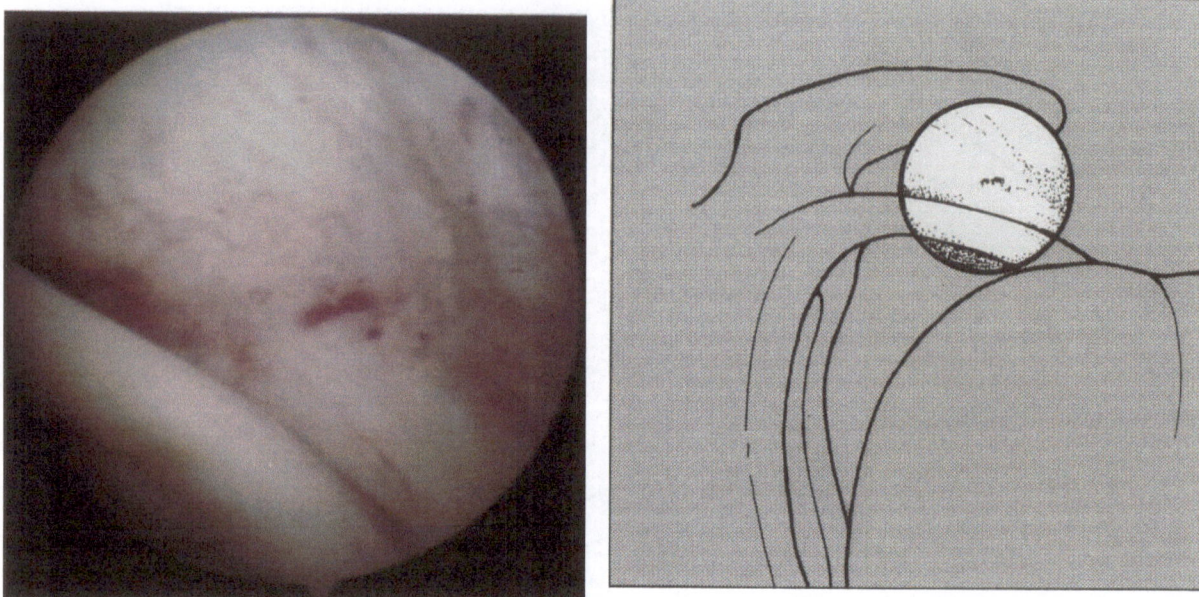

Fig. 58. Local synovitis of the rotator cuff: palpatory examination, possible bursoscopy indicated

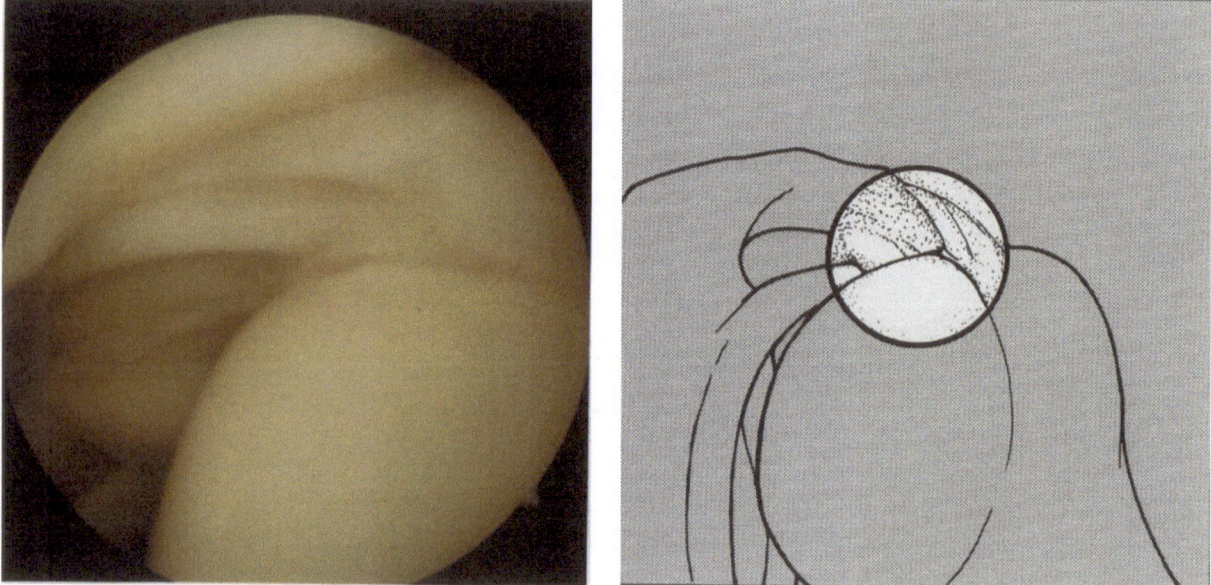

Fig. 59. Rotator cuff close to its attachment (infraspinatus tendon), zone without cartilage at the postero-lateral aspect of the humeral head (posterior synovial reflection)

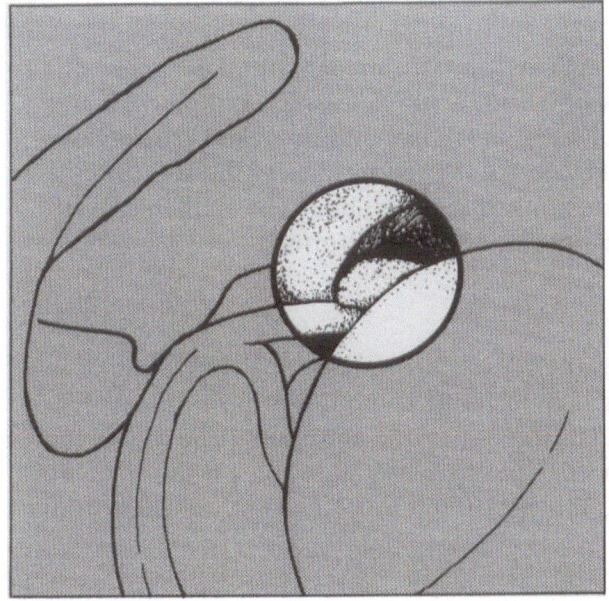 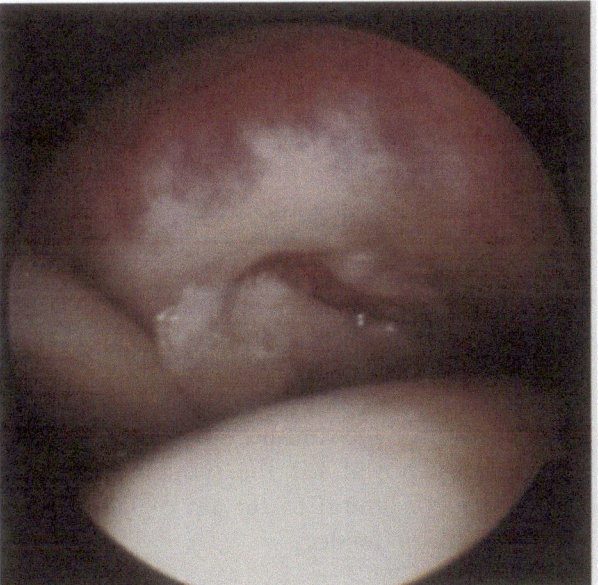

Fig. 60. Rupture of the rotator cuff near the attachment of the supraspinatus, synovitic changes in the surrounding area

Alternatively, arthroscopy can be performed with the patient in a half-sitting position (beach-chair position): the upper part of the operating table is raised and the patient is seated on a thick foam rubber wedge. The shoulder to be operated on projects above the upper edge of the operating table and is easily accessible. The major advantage of this position is that most surgical procedures in the shoulder can be carried out without changing the patient's position [12, 26].

Using a special elbow brace with the elbow in a right angle position not only allows the attachment of a traction cord but also enables the assistant surgeon to perform controlled rotatory movements of the patient's arm. These rotatory movements are required for the complete inspection of the rotator cuff and humeral head as well as for the functional examination of the anterior stabilizers [20]. For a solely diagnostic examination a traction weight of 3 or 5 kg is sufficient when the patient is in a lateral recumbent position and 2 to 3 kg in the beach-chair position. The arthroscopy is performed with the joint filled with fluid (Ringer's lactate solution or sugar solution), the flow is kept constant by hanging the fluid bag as high as possible or by using a pump.

Draping

After adequate skin preparation in the area of surgery, it should be isolated with adhesive waterproof drapes to ensure that the area of surgery is sterile and to prevent the patient from getting wet.

Instrumentation

The standard instrumentation for a diagnostic arthroscopy of the glenohumeral joint consists of an arthroscopic sheath, 5 mm, with a blunt trocar, a 30° wide-angle arthroscope and a 70° wide-angle scope, which is rarely used. Using a probe is mandatory and particularly important for evaluation of the labrum: a hooked probe is used to inspect the rotator cuff [19]. In addition, a rongeur, ligament forceps and hooked scissors should be available. With a powered shaver at hand a diagnostic bursoscopy can also be performed.

Portals

After outlining the landmarks, the sites of relevant portals are determined. For diagnostic arthroscopy of the glenohumeral joint, the standard posterior and anterior portals are used. The posterior incision lies 1.5 cm medial and 1 cm inferior to the acromial angle and is the obligatory portal for the scope. The incision for the standard anterior portal is made immediately lateral to the tip of the coracoid, the probe entering the joint cranial to the subscapularis tendon.

Arthroscopic examination

We recommend initial puncture and filling of the joint with a thin puncture needle using Ringer's solution (30 ml) for the less experienced. This enables determination of the plane of entry into the joint, ensures correct positioning of the cannula through aspiration of the joint and minimizes the danger of intraarticular injuries when inserting the arthroscopic sheath into the joint [11, 13].

With sufficient experience, a blunt trocar may be used alone and the initial puncture and filling may be dispensed with. After the skin incision has been made, all deeper structures are pushed aside with circular movements of the arthroscopic sheath. The surgeon's other hand lies on the front of the shoulder, the middle finger at the humeral head and the index finger at the coracoid. In this way, it is very easy to distinguish between the head of the humerus and the posterior rim of the socket through the pressure felt on the index or middle finger when advancing the arthroscopic sheath and trocar in the direction of the coracoid. The posterior edge of the socket can readily be explored with the blunt tip of the trocar, lateral to it the capsule can be identified as a solid but elastic structure. If the head of the humerus is distracted from the glenoid by the assistant surgeon using traction in the axilla, the capsule is tensed, and can be perforated with moderate but controlled exertion of force.

Only when the arthroscopic sheath and trocar is in the correct position will it be possible to advance it in the plane of the socket. A tightly rolled drape is placed in the axilla to serve as a fulcrum and further opens the joint space.

Now the trocar is replaced by the scope and the joint is filled with Ringer's solution. Often the arthroscope is inserted too far into the joint near the front wall of the shoulder which impedes scope orientation. After controlled withdrawal of the arthroscope, the long biceps tendon and humeral head are easily identified. It is advisable to place the camera at the scope in such a way that the plane of the socket corresponds with the perpendicular on the screen.

The probe, the use of which is mandatory, is introduced through the standard anterior portal. It is advanced through continuous rotation and should enter the shoulder joint at the upper edge of the subscapularis tendon. Probing of the glenoid labrum and rotator cuff is particularly necessary for arthroscopic examination of these structures.

Inspection of the glenohumeral joint should be performed in a complete and standardized manner: with the biceps tendon aiding orientation, we proceed to its origin at the upper pole of the glenoid, follow the anterior glenoid labrum and also evaluate the glenoid and the anterior wall of the shoulder. After inspecting the axillary recess, we move over the posterior labrum back to the origin of the biceps tendon. The use of a 70° scope is hardly ever necessary. Now we follow the biceps tendon in a distal direction to its entrance into the bicipital groove, turn the scope above the head of the humerus in the direction of the attachment of the rotator cuff and identify the area of the humeral head free of cartilage or a possible Hill-Sachs lesion. By turning the arthroscope and moving it in the horizontal plane while the upper arm of the patient is being rotated by the assistant, the rotator cuff can be surveyed in its entirety.

If no arthroscopic procedure or diagnostic bursoscopy is intended, the arthroscopy is completed after irrigation of the joint. Excess irrigation fluid is removed by suction, the arthroscope is removed, and a suction drain is placed through the sheath in case of intraarticular bleeding. The skin incisions are closed with single sutures and the arm is placed in a sling. Swelling of the shoulder due to accumulation of fluid in the soft tissues is harmless and is absorbed within about 24 hours. The patient is able to return to work within ten days of arthroscopy, depending on the primary pathology.

Glenoid labrum

The area of the cartilaginous surface of the humeral head, relative to that of the glenoid cavity is 3–4:1. This disproportion of the joint surfaces is partially compensated for by the glenoid labrum. This joint lip surrounds the bony glenoid in an annular fashion and is triangular when viewed in cross-section. The base of the labrum is fixed to the bony glenoid. The medial surface is attached to the joint capsule, mainly antero-inferiorly and posteriorly, while the free surface faces towards the joint (Figs. 37 and 38). In contrast to the situation during arthroscopy, the free surface of the labrum is normally in direct contact with the humeral head.

Often incorrectly described as cartilaginous, the labrum mainly consists of collagenous connective tissue: an inner circular fibrous ring with the biceps tendon radiating into it, and radially arranged outer fibers. Histologically, the labrum is fixed to the glenoid by specially orientated collagen fibres on the base of fibrocartilage [15]. Reeves has shown that this attachment is the weakest point of the anterior part of the joint in a young person during forced external rotation. This corresponds with the frequency of labral detachments, particularly at the anterior rim of the glenoid [22].

Fibrillation of the labrum is found in cases of anterior subluxation in combination with a loosening of the basal anchoring. When the instability persists, the marginal cartilage covering of the glenoid fossa also shows signs of abrasion. Often, however, the symptoms of the subluxation are caused by a separation of the labrum with its fibrous ring remaining intact. Depending on the direction of the initial trauma, that is to say, on forced abductions and external rotations, the separation may either be found antero-superiorly, in the area of the notch, antero-inferiorly, or there may even be a complete detachment.

Particularly in cases of prior dislocation, a complete detachment or a destruction of the labrum may be noted. When the labrum is absent it usually lies at the anterior neck of the glenoid, where it is functionless. In cases of repeated dislocation the anterior rim of the glenoid is often rounded off or eroded.

Depending on the location, different kinds of labrum detachments may be distinguished. Pathogenesis, symptoms and clinical relevance vary accordingly. An antero-inferior labrum detachment results from the typical dislocation manoeuvre of abduction-external rotation and is called a Bankart lesion (Fig. 39). An antero-superior separation of the glenoid labrum was found mainly in throwing athletes by Andrews (Figs. 40–42). He considered the cause to be extreme traction on the long biceps tendon in the third phase of throwing and the braking action of the forced elbow extension [3]. As the lesion progresses, superior portions of the glenoid and the attachment of the long head of the biceps to the glenoid labrum are affected, thereby forming a S.L.A.P. lesion (Superior Labrum, both Anterior and Posterior [27]). The joint lip may be detached in a hood-like manner and pulled cranially by the traction of the tendon, like a bucket handle (Fig. 43).

Evaluating the age of all these injuries is difficult and only possible indirectly. Bleeding spots at the site of rupture indicate a fresh lesion (Fig. 40). Frayed or rounded structures indicate chronic lesions.

If a patient with impingement symptoms is found to have vascular injection and basal loosening of the superior glenoid labrum at arthroscopy as well as increased vascularization or even synovitis of the adjacent biceps tendon and rotator cuff, it can be made a diagnosis of so-called secondary impingement (Fig. 44). An assumption can be made that the labrum damage described above allows superior migration of the head and subsequent impingement under the acromion and the coracoacromial ligament (see Chap. 6.3).

Anterior wall

The anterior portions of the joint capsule with its reinforcing ligaments and tendons is termed the anterior wall of the shoulder joint. At arthroscopy structures are visualized which are difficult to identify during open shoulder surgery [18] (Fig. 45). The capsule with its synovial and fibrous layers generally offers little resistance to the increased intraarticular pressure and bulges out, while the more substantial structures taut and more readily visible. The anatomy and functional significance of these structures becomes clear upon arthroscopy of the joint.

One landmark during examination of the anterior wall of the shoulder is the pronounced upper margin of the subscapularis tendon (Fig. 46). Coming into view at a right angle to the anterior rim of the glenoid, the tendon is seen to be running horizontally to the lesser tuberosity. It is separated from the interior of the joint by capsule only, which is very thin at this point.

The so-called reinforcing ligaments of the anterior shoulder joint capsule vary in their occurrence, course and shape; their identification and evaluation are, however, important for the performance of anterior arthroscopic stabilizing procedures.

The superior glenohumeral ligament arises with great variability at the superior neck of the scapula. It extends as a cord in a synovial sheath at an acute angle to the biceps tendon to its point of insertion at the anatomical neck proximal to the lesser tubercle. One branch embraces the biceps tendon from behind at its entrance into the bicipital groove. The ligament is always present, but probably of little functional significance.

The middle glenohumeral ligament, which is inconsistent in occurrence and shape, originates from the antero-superior rim of the socket. It crosses the subscapularis tendon in an infero-lateral direction, forming an obtuse angle and inserts into the anatomical neck of the humeral head. The distal portion of the ligament fuses with the subscapularis tendon, which has the same insertion.

The inferior glenohumeral ligament, originating from the glenoid labrum at the antero-inferior rim of the socket, is a well-defined fibrous plate with a thick superior border and inserts at the anatomical neck.

The latter two ligaments impede external rotation of the upper arm in various positions of abduction.

Between the superior and middle glenohumeral ligament the so-called upper anterior recess is found, which contains the subscapularis tendon. The entrance to this recess often contains loose bodies and is also known as Weitbrecht's foramen. The lower anterior recess is bounded by the middle glenohumeral ligament cranially and caudally by the inferior glenohumeral ligament. When the middle glenohumeral ligament is absent (seven percent of all cases) we then refer to the (great) anterior recess. More detailed descriptions of the variants of the anterior shoulder wall and their relationships to the adjacent bursae of the shoulder joint are given by DePalma, Hempfling, and Resch [9, 13, 14, 24].

If the arthroscope is turned downwards across the inferior portion of the socket, the axillary recess is found, which is wide in the healthy patient, bulging inferiorly (Fig. 47). It is the most common location of loose bodies. Inferiorly it is adjoined by the posterior circumflex humeral artery and axillary nerve. In the shoulder which is chronically restricted in movement, the capsule which forms the axillary recess is taut and the recess small. By withdrawing and rotating the scope the dorsal portion of the labrum can be seen and evaluations of its structure and firmness can be made with a probe (Fig. 48). Only in a few cases is an anterior portal required for the scope in order to inspect the posterior joint structures.

Glenoid cavity

The shoulder joint socket is a shallow hollow and has roughly the shape of an inverted comma. The longitudinal diameter runs parallel to the axis of the body. The transverse diameter is larger in its caudal than in its cranial portion, and the anterior rim is somewhat indented. This indentation is called the glenoid notch.

The articular cartilage is thinnest centrally, but this is hardly discernible at arthroscopy. Contusions of the glenohumeral joint alone may lead to bleeding or fractures of the cartilage, which, when they have been present for a long period of time, cannot be differentiated from cartilage softening or defects of a purely degenerative nature (Fig. 49).

However, we should differentiate signs of abrasion and erosions of the cartilage at the anterior rim of the socket, since these are commonly associated with lesions of the glenoid labrum, usually as a result of (repeated) glenohumeral subluxations or dislocations [20].

Biceps tendon

The tendon of the long head of the biceps, which is called "long biceps tendon" to simplify matters, is an eye-catcher after inserting the scope into the glenohumeral joint. It serves a landmark and starting point for arthroscopic examination. Originating from the supra-glenoid tubercle of the scapula, the biceps tendon is not only connected macroscopically but also histologically to the superior portion of the glenoid labrum [15]. It runs in an antero-su-perior direction obliquely across the joint and disappears into the funnel-shaped entrance of the bicipital groove. On the posterior side it is encircled by a branch of the superior gleno-humeral ligament [13] (Fig. 50).

When intraarticular pressure is at physiological levels, the rotator cuff rests against the biceps tendon, but at arthroscopy the pressure is elevated and the cuff bulges out as the joint fills with irrigating solution especially when the muscles are simultaneously relaxed.

Running intraarticularly, the biceps tendon normally shows little, if any vascularization (Fig. 51). Increased vascularization or even villonodular synovitis is, therefore, hardly ever an isolated occurrence in the sense of a "biceps tendinitis", but usually arises in concurrence with other pathologic processes such as in the course of an impingement syndrome (Fig. 52).

A lesion of the rotator cuff, especially when chronic, and also repeated glenohumeral subluxation may alter the adjacent biceps tendon.

Degeneration of the long biceps tendon, usually seen as fibrillation and thinning, is most often the result of rotator cuff pathology or an impingement syndrome (Figs. 53 and 54).

The final stage of these changes, rupture of the biceps tendon, is hardly ever an isolated occurrence but usually the result of a tear of the rotator cuff, existing for months or years [4]. In this case the moment of rupture is often undramatic and painless. The biceps tendon is sometimes fixed in the sulcus by its inflamed synovial sheath, which means that there is not always the characteristic muscle bulge. The site of rupture is most common where the tendon has the greatest curvature, that is to say, in the intertubercular groove, but it may also be found near the site of insertion or in its intraarticular course.

If the subscapularis tendon is partially torn near its insertion, the biceps tendon may be medially displaced from the groove in the sense of a subluxation or dislocation. In this case there is also the danger of rupture of the tendon.

Head of the humerus

The head of the humerus has the shape of a hemisphere. When entering the joint with the arthroscope it is a dominant feature along with the biceps tendon.

Arthroscopically, a maximum of one third of the cartilage-covered humeral head can be inspected at a time, a complete survey is only possible through rotation of the upper arm (arthroscopic elbow brace; see Chap. 3). Damage to the cartilage through traumatic contu-sion alone as well as degenerative changes are possible, as with the glenoid (Fig. 55).

The anatomical specificity of the dorsolateral zone without cartilage with the different degenerative changes at the insertion of the rotator cuff are described in the following section.

The Hill-Sachs lesion, which is to be differentiated from the lesions mentioned above, is one of the so-called secondary lesions which occur upon dislocation of the shoulder when the humeral head is caught at the antero-inferior rim of the socket. The radiodiagnostic term of Hill-Sachs lesion only includes the radiologically recognizable impressed fracture, situated dorso-laterally on the head of the humerus. By means of arthroscopy, equivalents to the Hill-Sachs lesion can be identified. The severity of the latter ranges from cartilage contusion to chondral fractures alone to deep osteochondral defects; all these lesions become rounded and smooth when in existence for longer periods (Fig. 56). This area can be inspected arthroscopically through retraction of the arthroscope and simultaneous external rotation of the upper arm by the assistant. Possible entrapment of the Hill-Sachs lesion at the anterior rim of the socket and thus the probability of a recurrent dislocation can be evaluated in the course of such a dynamic test [11]. The secondary changes at the anterior rim of the socket (labrum disruption, possible bony Bankart lesion) and the state of the anterior wall of the capsule can also be assessed.

Rotator cuff

The rotator cuff arthroscopically consists of the tendons of the supraspinatus, the infraspinatus, and the teres minor muscles. The tendon of the subscapularis muscle is part of the anterior wall of the shoulder and has been described above. The coracohumeral ligament, which runs from the base of the coracoid to the two tuberosities, and which closes the gap between the supraspinatus and the subscapularis muscle, cannot usually be seen arthroscopically.

For arthroscopic evaluation of the rotator cuff, the rolled drape, placed in the axilla, is removed to relax the tendons. After the inspection of the long biceps tendon the scope is slowly turned towards the humeral head and the rotator cuff is identified in its lateral course near its insertion. When the arthroscope is rotated in the horizontal plane (in relation to the patient's body) and the humeral head externally rotated by the assistant (elbow brace) the tendons can be seen in their entirety.

Viewed intraarticularly, the rotator cuff is only covered by the superiorly thin, relatively avascular joint capsule and cannot be separated from it. The rotator cuff is silvery white and shiny, its longitudinal fibres readily recognizable (Fig. 57). Any change of the synovia, such as locally increased vascularization or even villonodular synovitis, is always an indication of damage to the tendon and requires meticulous palpation with a probe, and in case of a negative finding a bursoscopy (Fig. 58). The rotator cuff inserts at the anatomical neck of the humeral head in the region of the two tuberosities at the margin of the cartilage covering the head. Postero-laterally, the insertion retreats up to 10 mm from the margin of the cartilage, thus creating a cartilage-free zone, which DePalma calls the "sulcus". This area is normally covered by synovium, which forms a fold at the insertion of the tendon and which extends to the cartilage border and has a longitudinally folded shape. In the course of a lifetime changes take place here, ranging from synovial defects to degenerative arthritic serrations at the margins. Care must be taken not to confuse these changes with a Hill-Sachs lesion [18] (Fig. 59).

If the rotator cuff shows the synovial changes mentioned above, palpation often reveals incomplete ruptures on the synovial aspect. These cannot normally be detected arthrographically because they are covered. Intratendinous calcium deposits may, however, also lead to synovial reactions (see Chap. 5). Partial tears of the rotator cuff which are not covered show fibrous, degenerative, frayed or rounded, swollen edges depending on the age of the lesion [19]. This also applies to a complete tear, which gives a view of the bursa or the undersurface of the acromion (Fig. 60). These complete tears, however, are usually diagnosed sonographically or at least arthrographically.

Incomplete tears of the acromial aspect of the rotator cuff cannot be diagnosed from the glenohumeral joint, which means that a complete endoscopic diagnosis of the rotator cuff is only possible with a subsequent bursoscopy.

References

1. Altchek DW, Warren RF, Skyhar MJ (1990) Shoulder arthroscopy. In: Rockwood CA Jr, Matsen MA III (eds) The shoulder. WB Saunders, Philadelphia, pp 258–277

2. Andrews JR (1984) Arthroscopy of the shoulder: technique and normal anatomy. Am J Sports Med 12:1–7

3. Andrews JR, Carson WG, McLeod WD (1985) Glenoid labrum tears related to the long head of the biceps. Am J Sports Med 13:337–341

4. Apoil A (1977) Le syndrome, dit "le rupture de la coiffe des rotateurs de l'epaule". Rev Chir Orthop 63:145

5. Beck E (1987) Bildgebende Verfahren an der Schulter. In: Gächter A (ed) Arthroskopie der Schulter. Enke, Stuttgart, pp 14–16 [Hofer H, Glinz W (eds) Fortschritte in der Arthroskopie, vol 3]

6. Benedetto KP, Glötzer W, Künzel KH (1987) Anatomische Grundlagen für die Arthroskopie des Schultergelenkes. In: Gächter A (ed) Arthroskopie der Schulter. Enke, Stuttgart, pp 17–20 [Hofer H, Glinz W (eds) Fortschritte in der Arthroskopie, vol 3]

7. Blachut PA, Day B (1989) Arthroscopic anatomy of the shoulder. J Arthrosc Relat Surg 5:1–10

8. Cofield RH (1983) Arthroscopy of the shoulder. Mayo Clinic Proc 58:501–508

9. DePalma AF (1983) Surgery of the shoulder. JB Lippincott, Philadelphia

10. Fick R (1904) Handbuch der Anatomie und Mechanik der Gelenke. Fischer, Jena

11. Gächter A, Seelig W (1988) Schulterarthroskopie. Arthroskopie 1:162–170

12. Habermeyer P, Krueger P, Schweiberer L (1990) Schulterchirurgie. Urban & Schwarzenberg, Wien

13. Hempfling H (1987) Farbatlas der Arthroskopie großer Gelenke. G Fischer, Stuttgart

14. Hempfling H (1989) Einführung in die Arthroskopie. G Fischer, Stuttgart

15. Hertz H, Weinstabl R, Grundschober F, Orthner F (1986) Zur makroskopischen und mikroskopischen Anatomie der Schultergelenkspfanne und des Limbus glenoidalis. Acta Anat 125:96–100

16. Hertz H (1987) Schulterarthroskopie nach frischer traumatischer Schulterluxation. In: Gächter A (ed) Arthroskopie der Schulter. Enke, Stuttgart, pp 41–43 [Hofer H, Glinz W (eds) Fortschritte in der Arthroskopie, vol 3]

17. Jakob RP, Stäubli HU (1987) Stellenwert der Schulterarthroskopie. In: Gächter A (ed) Arthroskopie der Schulter. Enke, Stuttgart, pp 44–56 [Hofer H, Glinz W (eds) Fortschritte in der Arthroskopie, vol 3]

18. Johnson LL (1987) The shoulder joint. Clin Orthop 223:113–125

19. Lilleby H (1984) Shoulder arthroscopy. Acta Orthop Scand 55:561–566

20. McGlynn FJ, Caspari RB (1984) Arthroscopic findings in the subluxating shoulder. Clin Orthop 183:173–178
21. Ogilvie-Harris DJ, Wiley AM (1986) Arthroscopic surgery of the shoulder. J Bone Joint Surg [Br] 68:201–207
22. Reeves B (1968) Experiments on the tensile strength of the anterior capsular structures of the shoulder in man. J Bone Joint Surg [Br] 55:858
23. Resch H, Beck E (eds) (1988) Praktische Chirurgie des Schultergelenkes. Frohnweiler, Innsbruck
24. Resch H (1989) Die vordere Instabilität des Schultergelenkes. Hefte Unfallheilk 202:115–163
25. Seiler H, Neumann K, Muhr G (1984) Die Arthroskopie des Schultergelenkes. Unfallheilkunde 87:73–77
26. Skyhar MJ, Altchek DW, Warren RF, Wickiewicz TL, O'Brien SJ (1988) Shoulder arthroscopy with the patient in beach-chair position. Arthroscopy 4:256–259
27. Snyder SJ, Kartel RP, DelPizzo W, Ferkel RD, Freedman MJ (1990) S.L.A.P. lesions of the shoulder. Arthroscopy 6:274–279
28. Winnie AP (1970) Interscalene brachial plexus block. Anesth Analg 49:455

5 Diagnostic bursoscopy

G. Sperner, H. Resch, and K. Golser

Indications

Impingement syndrome

Impingement of the shoulder is a bottle-neck syndrome in the subacromial space. For a variety of reasons, the normally smooth glide of the rotator cuff between humeral head and acromion is disturbed (e.g., tendon rupture, subacromial bursitis, inflammatory swelling of the tendon, constriction of the subacromial space due to osteophytes, large calcareous deposits in the tendon, displaced fractures of the greater tuberosity, etc.).

Pathological changes in the subacromial space can usually be detected in the course of a clinical examination. We have various diagnostic techniques at our disposal for this purpose.

1. Clinical tests.   A large range of such tests have been described in literature; a few very specific tests are usually sufficient. It is not until we have excluded an injury to the acromio-clavicular joint as well as an instability of the glenohumeral joint that the subacromial space is examined clinically [12].

- Supraspinatus test as described by Jobe (Fig. 61). The arm is extended in 90° of abduction and is then elevated against resistance exerted by the examiner. This examination is performed in both internal and external rotation. If these movements are accompanied by pain, we may refer to a bottle-neck syndrome in the broadest sense.
- Horizontal adduction test (Fig. 62). The arm of the injured shoulder is moved towards the healthy one. After having excluded a lesion of the AC joint, which also shows a positive test, this test is an excellent method for detection of an impingement syndrome.
- "Tail coat pocket grip" (Fig. 63). By passive combined adduction, internal rotation and extension of the arm a sharp pain is provoked.
- Apprehension test (Fig. 64). The shoulder is moved passively into maximum external rotation in abduction and forward pressure is applied to the posterior aspect of the humeral head. The arm is in 90° of abduction. If this test is positive in combination with the others mentioned above, a so-called instability impingement (secondary impingement) can be diagnosed (see below). If only the apprehension test is positive, we are probably dealing with a purely anterior instability.
- LA-test (Fig. 65). 3–5 ml of a local anesthetic is injected into the subacromial space. If the pain disappears after a few minutes, we may conclude that there are pathological changes in the subacromial space.

2. X-rays.   Radiographs of the shoulder in two planes (ap and axial) are routinely performed on every patient. For a more detailed visualization of the subacromial space we perform an additional lateral view (outlet view) of the scapula [1].

– Sclerosis and cyst formation on the undersurface of the acromion and on the greater tuberosity. These are an indication of damage to the tendon due to long-term mechanical irritation.
– Subacromial osteophyte. Degenerative spur on the inferior acromial surface, which eventually leads to a rupture of the tendon due to its mechanical irritation. This spur can be evaluated in detail by means of a radiograph as described by Rockwood (the central beam is angled 30° inferiorly in the a.p. X-ray) or through the outlet view of the scapula, which we prefer (Fig. 66) [6].
– Superior migration of the humeral head. This is the expression of an extensive tear of the rotator cuff. In addition, atrophic changes of the bone can often be seen when the rotator cuff tear is chronic as well as degenerative arthritis of the glenohumeral joint of varied intensity or even a "cuff arthropathy" as described by Neer [7].
– Calcifying tendinitis. Calcareous deposits of varied size are mostly found in the region of the supra- or infraspinatus tendons. For better localization, additional radiographs with the arm in 60° of internal or external rotation are helpful.
– Degenerative arthritis of the acromio-clavicular joint. It is important diagnostically to differentiate this problem from possible pathologic changes in the subacromial space.

3. Ultrasound.   Sonographic investigation of the shoulder joint is carried out routinely in cases of clinically suspected diseases or injuries of the rotator cuff (Fig. 67) [2, 9, 11].

– Complete rupture. A complete full-thickness tear of the tendon can be diagnosed very accurately with sonography.
– Incomplete rupture. An incomplete tear of the tendon on the acromial side can only be detected sonographically if the rupture has a concave shape and comprises about half of the thickness of the tendon. Incomplete ruptures on the synovial side are hardly discernible on sonography; we therefore recommend an additional arthrogram of the glenohumeral joint.
– Calcifying tendinitis. These calcareous deposits, which are very homogeneous in their consistence, are noted as areas which produce very distinct echoes and have sonographic shadows behind them.
– Inflammatory swelling of the tendon. This is easily discerned by measuring and comparing its thickness with that of the contralateral tendon assuming the latter is healthy.
– Thickening of the bursa. When comparing it with the healthy side, a swollen, thickened subacromial and/or subdeltoid bursa may be seen as an expression of an increased accumulation of liquid due to inflammation. On ultrasound, a bandlike area with hardly any echo can be seen in the bursal area.

These methods of examination demonstrate that the causes of the bottle-neck syndrome are very diverse. Impingement in the broadest sense is to be understood as a term for changes and/or constrictions in the subacromial space which are triggered off by very different pathogenic mechanisms.

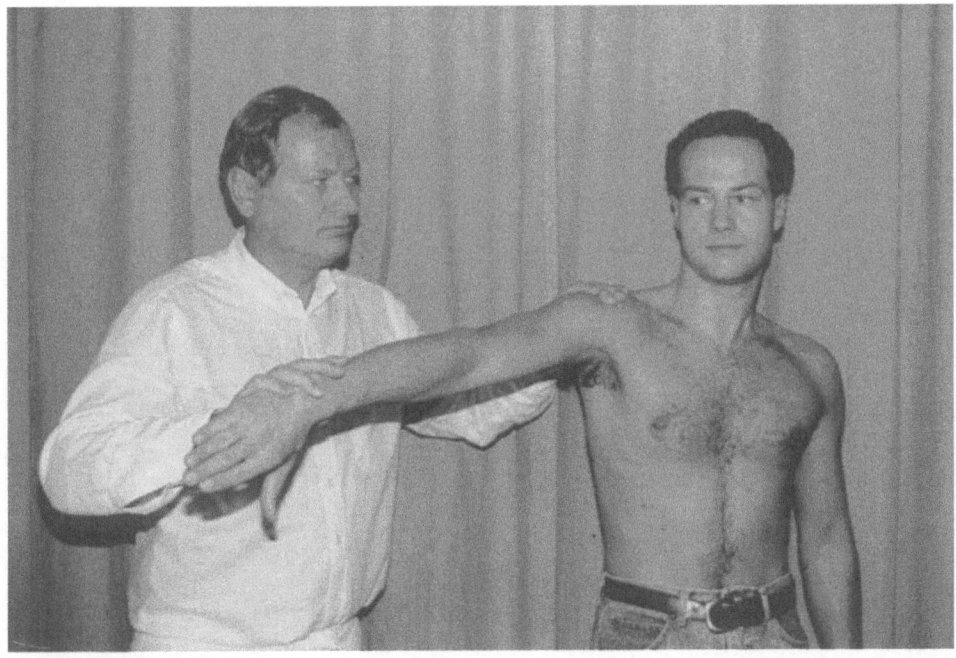

Fig. 61. Supraspinatus test as described by Jobe

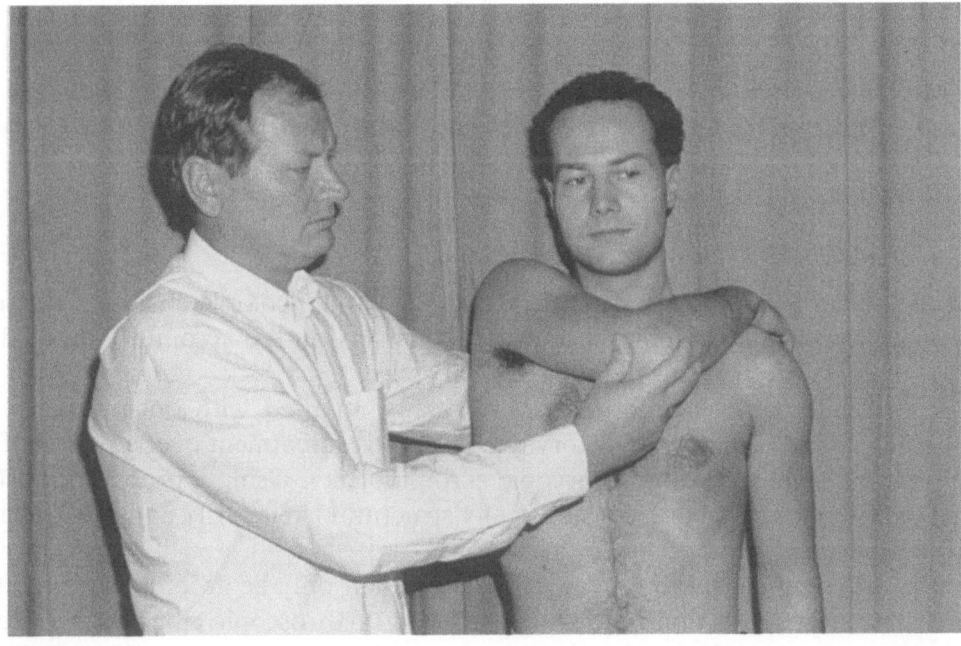

Fig. 62. Horizontal adduction test (cross body test)

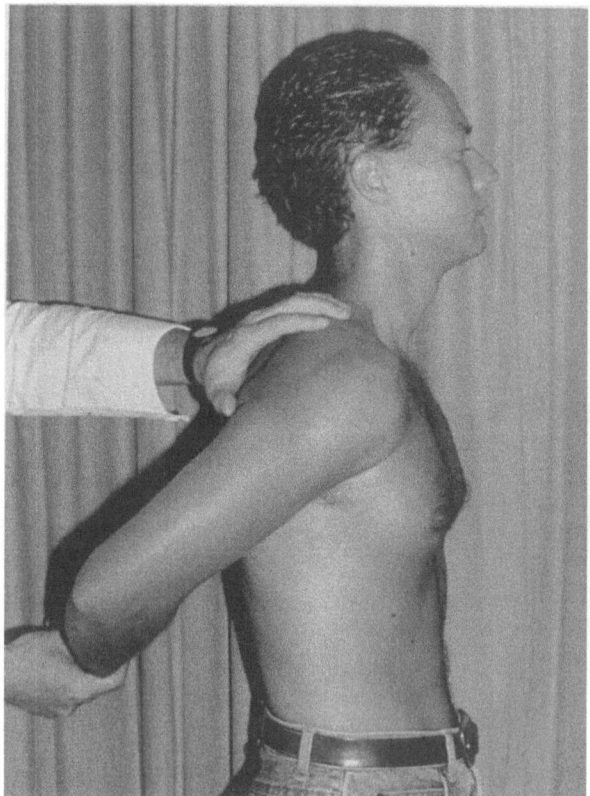 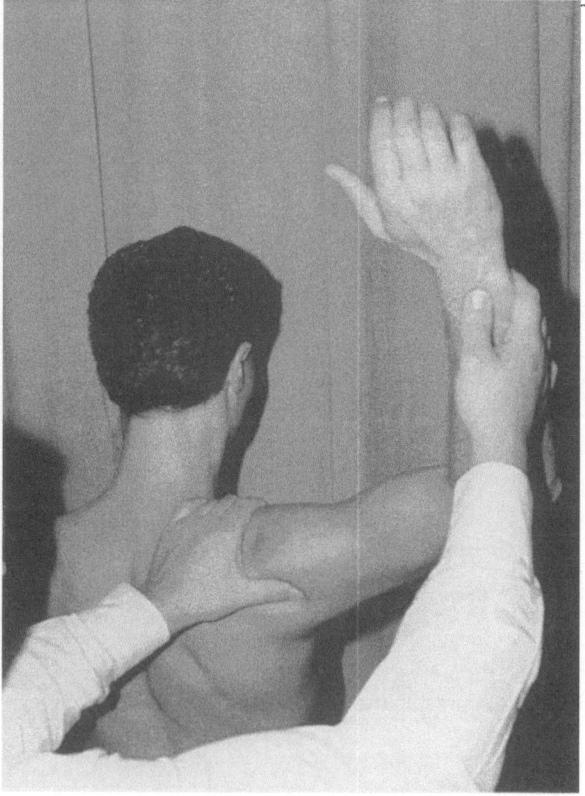

Fig. 63. "Tail coat pocket grip"   **Fig. 64.** Apprehension test

If conservative treatment is not successful, an arthroscopic subacromial decompression is carried out (see Chap. 7.1).

Incomplete ruptures

In accordance with the definition, complete and incomplete tears of the rotatur cuff lead to impingement symptoms since the frayed parts on the acromial side of the tendon hamper smooth movement in the subacromial space.

While complete ruptures are normally repaired with open surgical techniques, small incomplete ruptures, refractory to conservative treatment over a period of at least 6 months, can be managed with bursoscopic acromioplasty. Using a probe, the surface of the rotator cuff is palpated in order to detect any structural irregularity and/or fibrillation of the tendon tissue.

A complete survey of the whole bursa can only be accomplished by additional external and internal rotation of the humeral head (arthroscopic elbow brace; see Chap. 3). Due to the convexity of the subacromial space to be viewed, incomplete ruptures on the acromial side are best evaluated when they are not located near the attachment of the tendon but at its

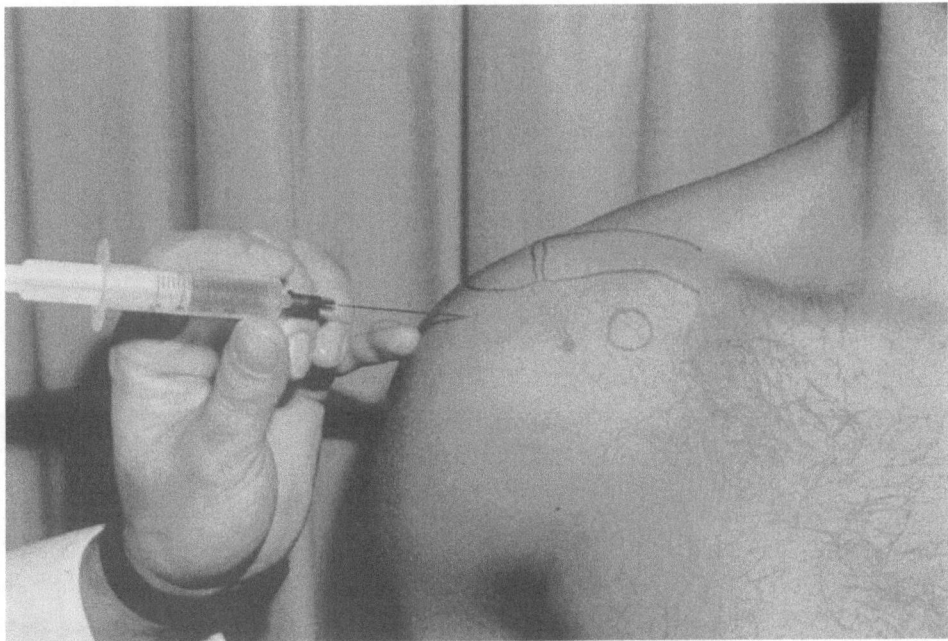

Fig. 65. LA-test (impingement-test according to Neer)

center. Incomplete lesions on the synovial side are not discernible bursoscopically, they should, however, already have been diagnosed by the arthroscopy of the glenohumeral joint conducted immediately before.

Calcifying tendinitis

Smaller deposits are usually asymptomatic, while larger deposits lead to a mechanical impingement because of the protrusion of the tendon. In the course of an acute inflammation the calcific tendinitis may suddenly disappear or dissolve. In this case the patients will complain of a sharp throbbing pain which normally lasts for five to seven days. Neither active nor passive movement is possible at this stage. Conservative measures such as rest, local cryotherapy, antiinflammatory medication and possibly a subacromial cortisone injection will help the acute symptoms subside more quickly. Depending on the size of the remaining calcareous deposit, chronic impingement-like pains may persist, but the symptoms may also resolve completely.

Radiologically, the extent of the calcareous deposit can be determined exactly. The localization is important for preoperative planning as smaller deposits are often embedded in the tendon, and therefore hard to discern bursoscopically. Normally they need not be treated. Larger deposits which touch the surface or protrude are easily detected on bursoscopy. They are noted to be pale-spotted, sometimes shiny plaques.

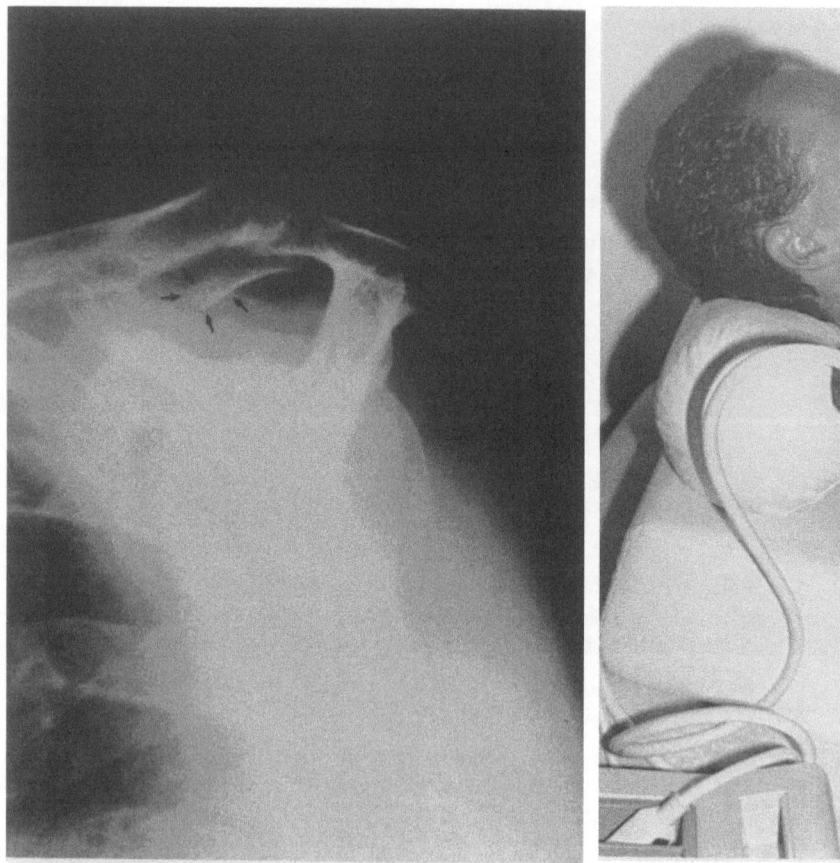
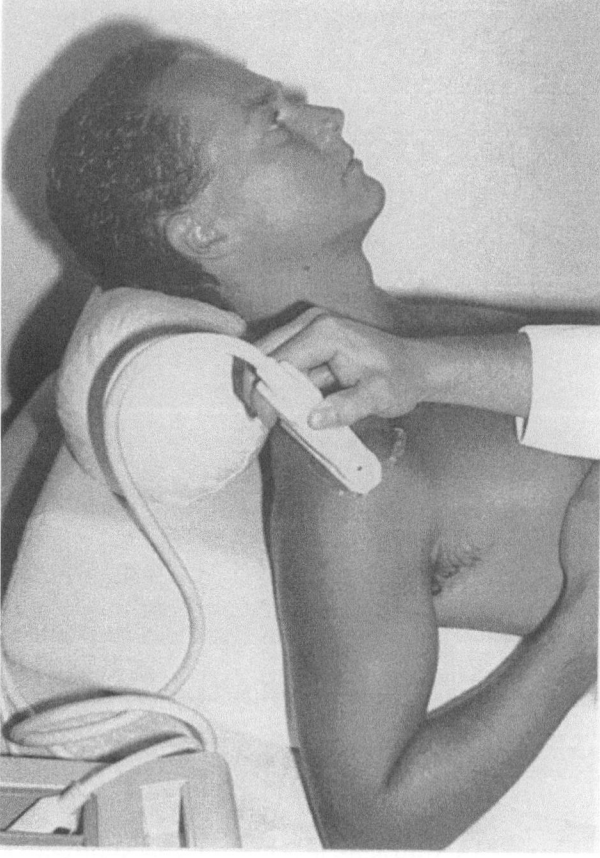

Fig. 66   Fig. 67

Fig. 66. Y-projection of the scapula: large osteophyte spur (arrows) which arises from the inferior acromial surface and constricts the subacromial space (and the rotator cuff)

Fig. 67. Positioning for ultrasonographic examination of the rotator cuff: upper part of the body slightly elevated, arm extended, adducted and slightly rotated internally; thus the supraspinatus tendon lies lateral to the acromion and the infraspinatus tendon anterior to it, ensuring good exposure for sonography, 7.5 MHz linear transducer used

The consistency of these deposits is diverse, ranging from a milky liquid to hard crumbly material. Liquid deposits are opened bursoscopically by scratching them with the probe, the calcareous content flows into the bursa and is removed by irrigation. If the consistency is viscous, the probe is used to squeeze the deposit and the contents expressed like toothpaste (see Chap. 7.2).

Secondary impingement

C. S. Neer believes that impingement syndrome always arises from the roof of the shoulder [7]. In contrast to this, patients with impingement syndromes often show changes to the

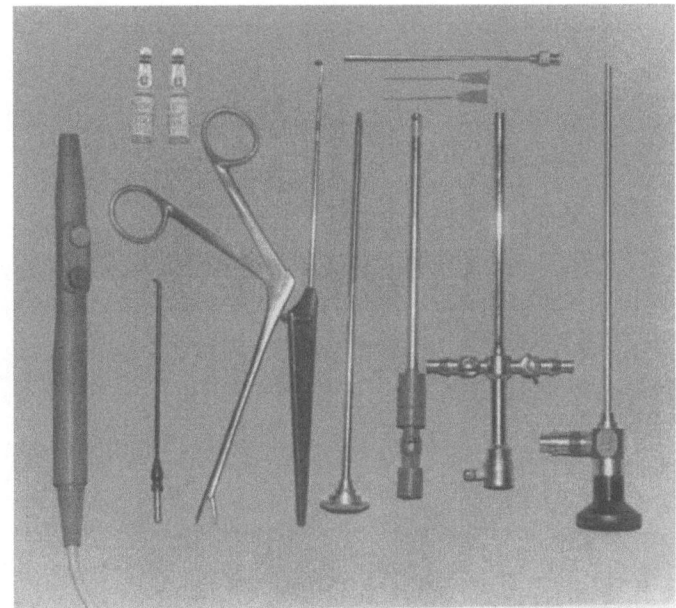

Fig. 68. Instrumentation for diagnostic bursoscopy (right to left): 30° wide-angle scope, sheath, shaver (synovial resector or full radius resector), blunt trocar, probe, rongeur, diathermy knife (completely isolated except for tip) with handle; above: cushing cannula, injection needles, 2 ampoules of ornithine-vasopressin

glenohumeral joint without any changes to the roof of the shoulder. In accordance with Paulos [10], we designate all impingement syndromes which do not arise from the roof of the shoulder as "secondary impingement syndrome", since they obviously stem from other causes.

Arthroscopic examination of patients with impingement syndromes commonly reveals the following findings.

- Local synovitis. This is noted as an increased injection of vessels with varying extension into the antero-superior portion of the joint. The origin of the biceps tendon is almost always involved as well as the superior portion of the labrum. In some very marked cases the inflammatory reddening spreads to the antero-superior synovia (synovial portion of the rotator cuff).
- Detachment of the antero-superior labrum. This detachment, termed as Andrews lesion, may extend as far as the glenoid notch. Sometimes the glenoid labrum is detached in a hoodlike manner from antero-superior to postero-superior along the glenoid rim with a disrupted origin of the biceps tendon. This is termed a S.L.A.P.-lesion (superior labrum both anterior and posterior lesion) [13]. One or the other of these lesions is found in many patients with impingement syndromes.

We believe that there is an increased upward and/or anterosuperior translation of the humeral head or even collison with the roof of the shoulder when the findings mentioned above are present. Thus, the subacromial space is constricted and a bottle-neck syndrome ensues. Multidirectional instabilities also show these findings but usually without any detachment of the labrum. Bursoscopically, an unremarkable subacromial space is noted, the

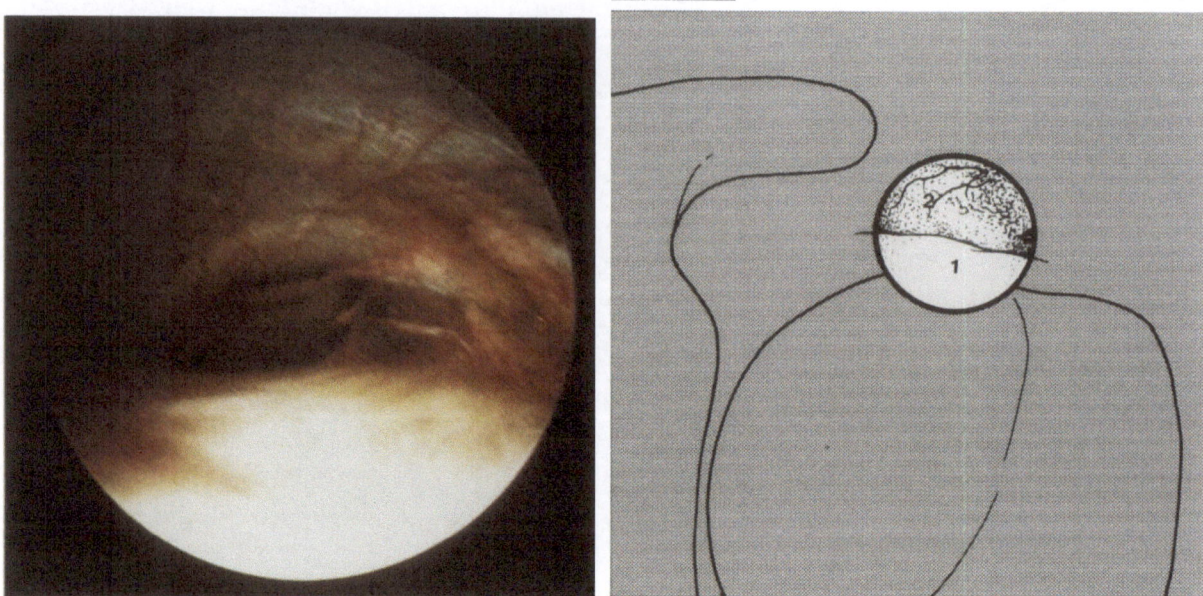

Fig. 69. Posterior view of subacromial bursa: smooth, intact tendon surface (*1*), in the background bursal roof (*2*) with slightly increased injection of vessels

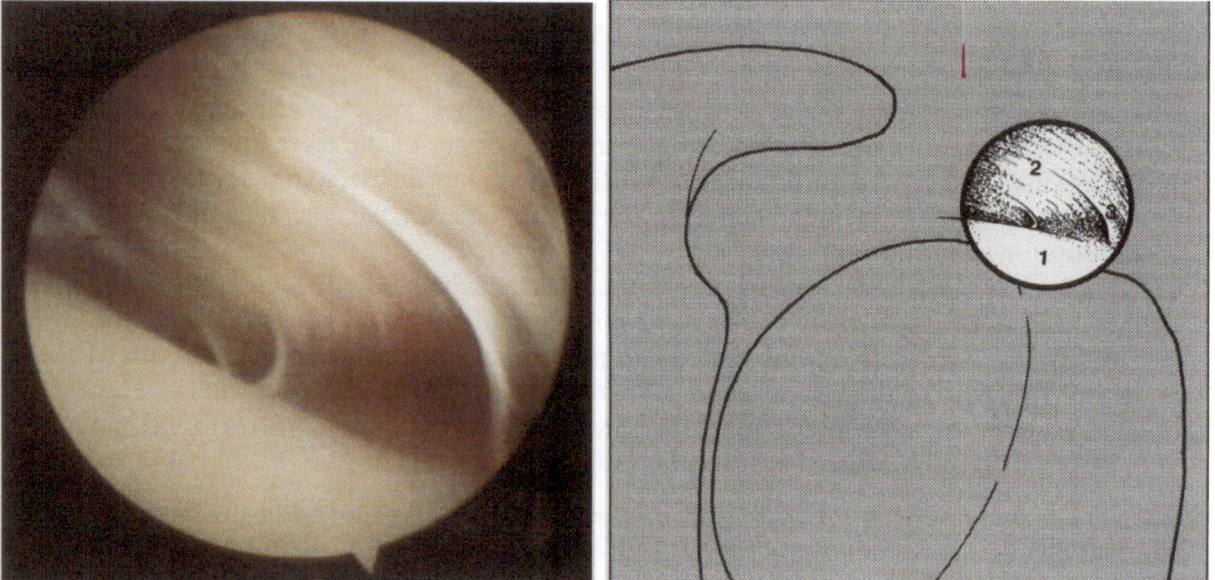

Fig. 70. In the front lies the intact acromial part of the surface of the rotator cuff (*1*), laterally and/or antero-laterally the bursa is noted to be bounded by septae (*2*); in between slight synovitic reddening

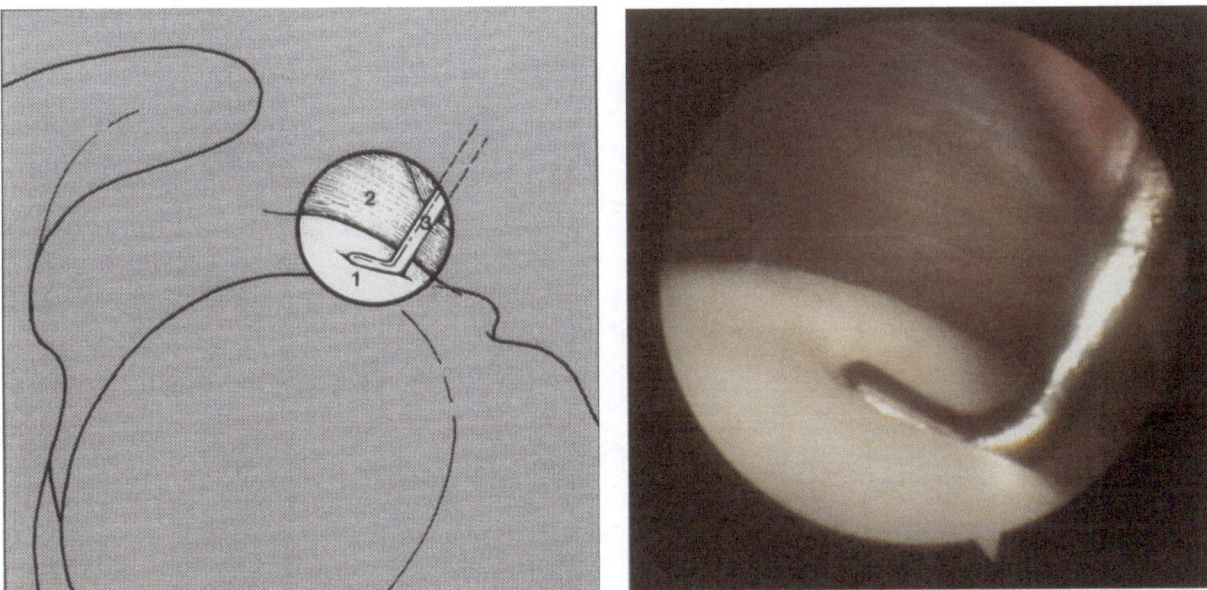

Fig. 71. Same patient as in Fig. 70. Palpation of the tendon surface with a probe inserted through the lateral portal (*3*) in order to detect any calcareous deposits or fibrillation of the rotator cuff. Simultaneous external and internal rotation of the humeral head allows visualization of the entire rotator cuff (*1*); in the background and above: roof of bursa (*2*)

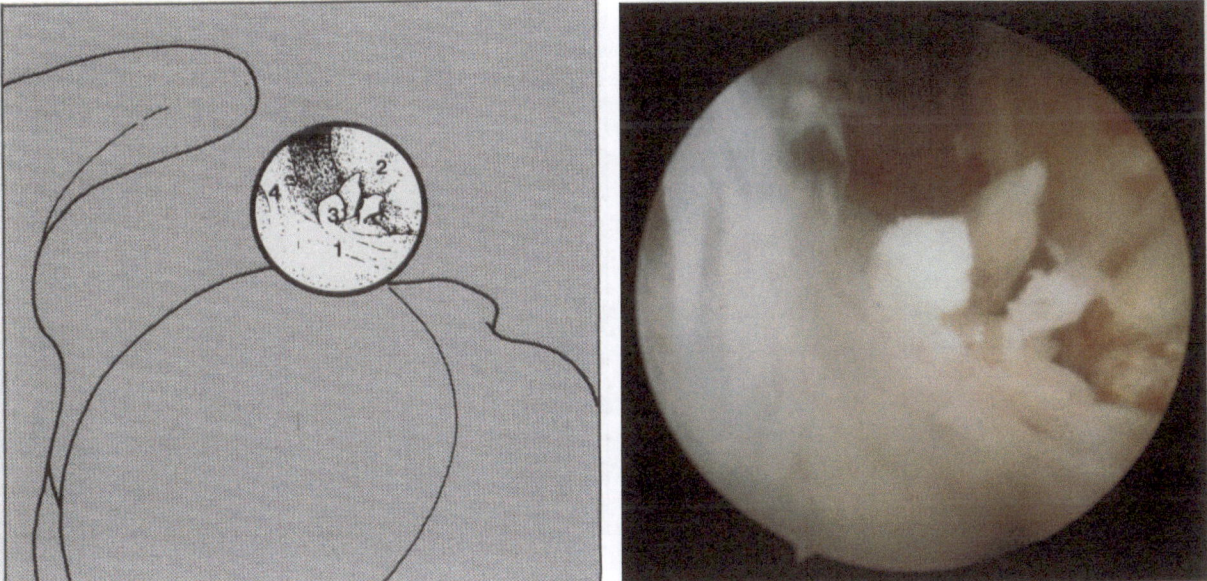

Fig. 72. Scratching and opening the surface of the tendon (*1*) to evacuate the calcareous deposit, calcium (*3*) (crumbly consistency) flows into subacromial space (*2*); thin bursa tissue (*4*)

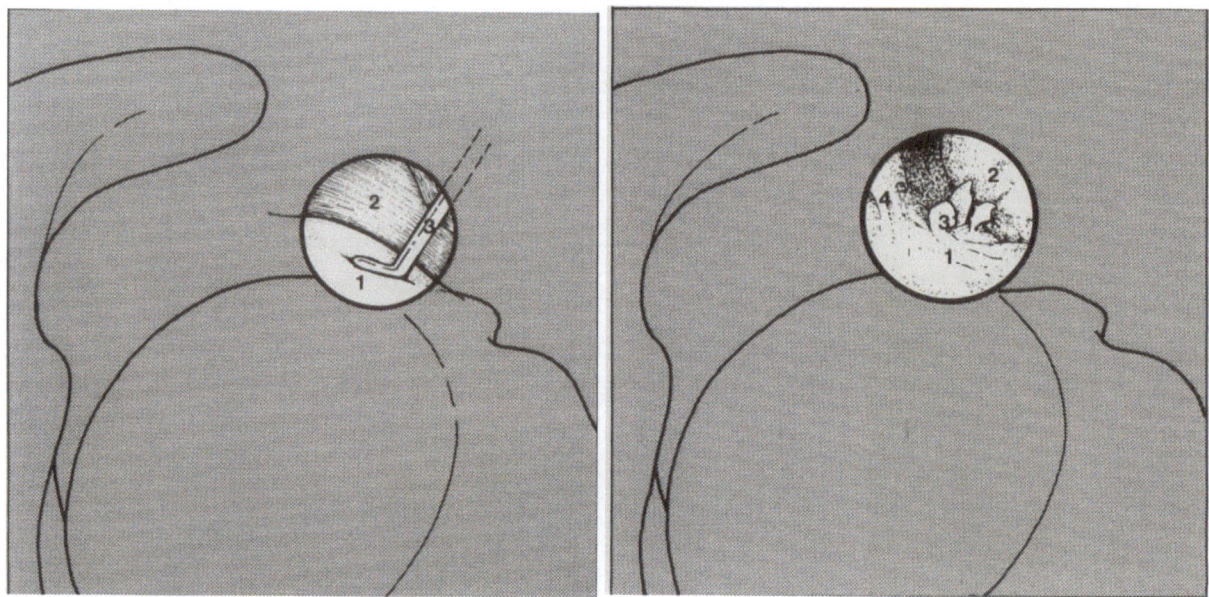

Fig. 73. Palpation of the surface of the rotator cuff (*1*) with the probe (*3*) to detect any ruptures on the acromial side (*2*)

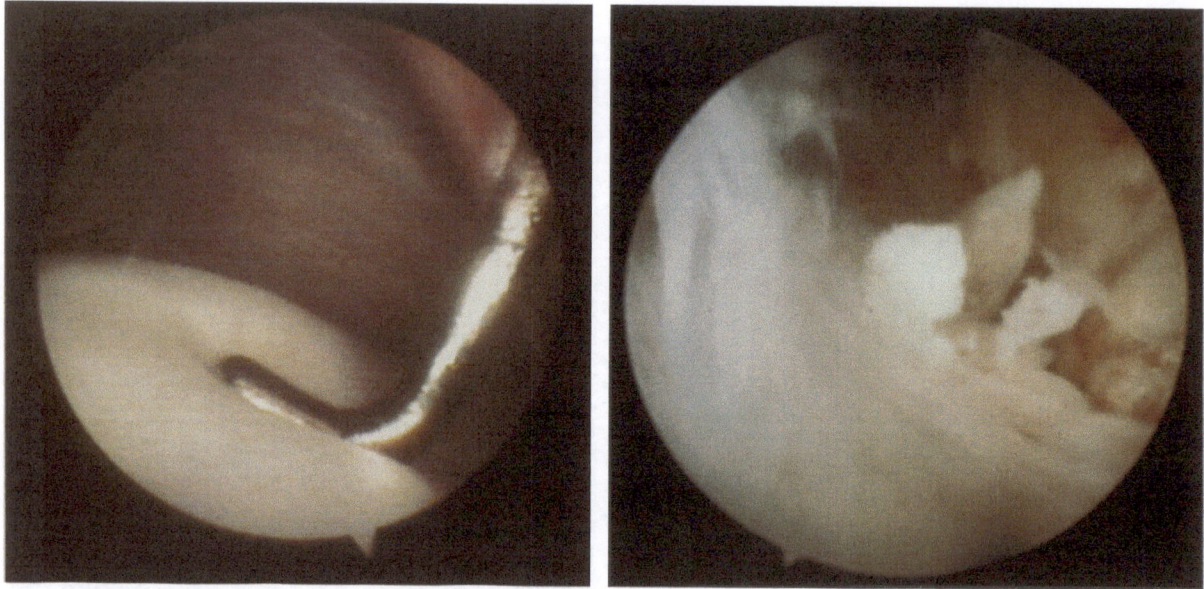

Fig. 74. Complete rupture of the rotator cuff (*2*). View from subacromial space (*3*) through ruptured tendon into the glenohumeral joint. Below right: cartilage covering of the humeral head (*1*); medially (below left): part of the long biceps tendon (*4*)

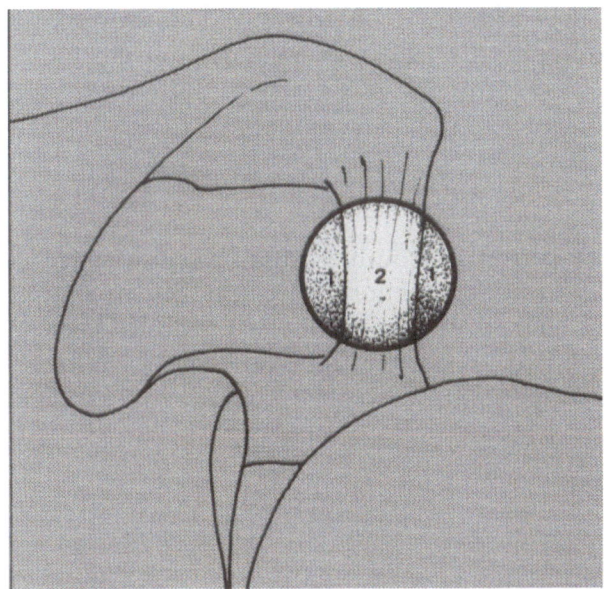
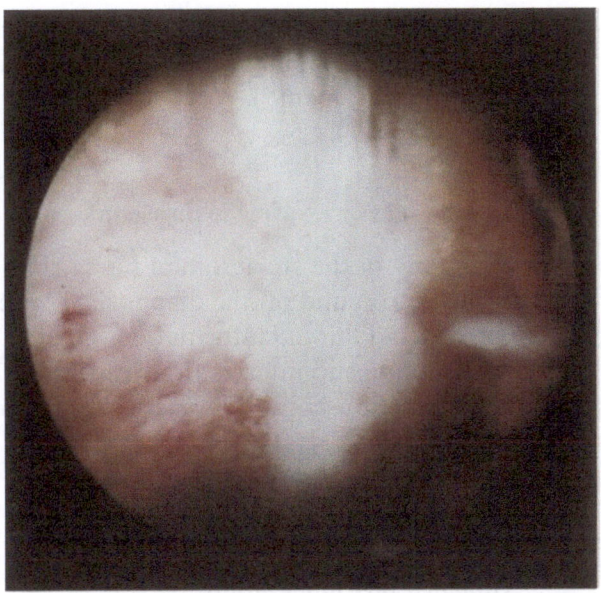

Fig. 75. To complete the diagnostic bursoscopy, the scope is turned 180°. View directed forwards and upwards. Starting from the anterior edge of the acromion, the coracoacromial ligament, which runs in an antero-medial direction, is located (2). Shaving of the surrounding bursal tissue (1) allows better visualization of the whole ligament

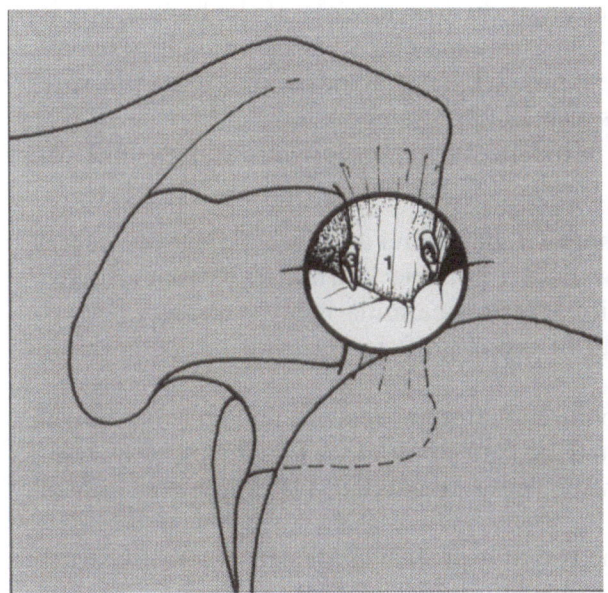
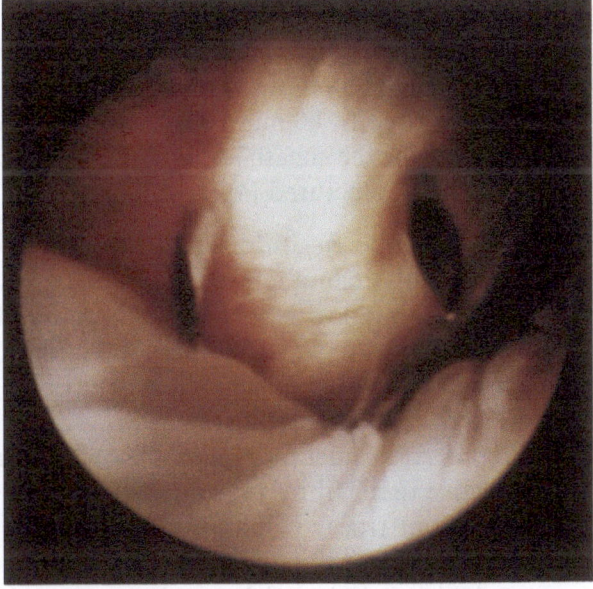

Fig. 76. Delineation of the width of the coracoacromial ligament (1) by percutaneous insertion of needles (3); surrounding bursal tissue (2)

rotatur cuff is mostly undamaged on the bursal side. Furthermore, hardly any changes to the bony roof of the shoulder are detectable radiographically (sclerosis, osteophytes, etc. = "primary impingement").

Routine measures after arthroscopy

A bursoscopy of the subacromial bursa should be performed routinely after every shoulder arthroscopy to round off the diagnosis. Especially when the diagnosis is unclear, bursoscopy may provide additional information. Operatively, there is little additional expenditure since in purely diagnostic interventions only the sheath is changed, the same posterior portal is used as for arthroscopy. The instruments are also the same.

Instruments

Standard instrumentation

Arthroscopy as well as bursoscopy are performed exclusively in a liquid environment and electrolyte (Ringer's lactate) or sugar solutions (Resectal) are used. Two ampules of 1 ml POR 8 (ornithine-vasopressin) each diluted to 20 ml may be injected into the subacromial space (especially in the direction of the acromial branch of the thoracoacromial artery) immediately after the preparation and draping. Through local vasoconstriction, better control of bleeding is achieved and thus a good view guaranteed. Furthermore, the bursa is distended, which greatly facilitates the introduction of the instruments. If the bursoscopy is performed under general anesthesia, obstructive bleeding may be avoided by slightly reducing the arterial blood pressure. In patients without any risk factors, the mean arterial pressure can be lowered to 80 mm Hg (for more details, see Chaps. 2 and 3).

Except for the sheath, all instruments used in diagnostic bursoscopy are routine and not specially manufactured [4] (Fig. 68).

- Arthroscope. In contrast to arthroscopy, where a 5 mm round arthroscope is used, we use a specially manufactured 6.5 mm high-flow sheath (Andre, Dornbirn) for bursoscopy. Thus, the inflow is increased and an additional inflow-cannula is not necessary.
- A 30° wide-angle scope illuminates the field of vision sufficiently, a 70° scope is rarely needed as a supplementary instrument.
- Trocar. When inserting the arthroscope into the subacromial space, a few very thin bursal septae are sometimes incompletely perforated, and an optimal view is impaired by connective tissue fibres in front of the scope. In such cases, medial and lateral movements of the blunt trocar will improve the view.
- Probe. As with arthroscopy of the knee, the use of a probe is indispensable. Any structural irregularity of the rotator cuff such as fibrillation, partial tears and protrusions of the tendon caused by calcareous deposits can be felt with the probe. In cases of bursitis, the probe is also used to push septa-like connective tissue layers aside, in order to improve the view.

- Rongeur. This instrument, normally used in ENT surgery, is ideally suited for the endoscopic removal of floating soft tissue obstructing the view. These forceps are absolutely indispensable for diagnostic as well as therapeutic interventions and should be part of every arthroscopic set.
- Shaver. A shaver with infinitely variable speed and a suction device is essential not only for therapeutic but also for purely diagnostic bursoscopy. It allows clear visualization of the subacromial space by sucking and shaving off strands of connective tissue which hang in front of the arthroscope. When performing subacromial decompression, these instruments are mainly used for the removal of ligamentous and periosteal tissue from the inferior surface of the acromion as well as for bony resection (see Chap. 7.1).

Supplementary instrumentation

A few additional instruments are useful for diagnostic bursoscopy, even though they do not belong to the essential basic equipment. After skin preparation and draping, the landmarks (acromion, AC joint with lateral clavicle, coracoid tip, coracoacromial ligament) are outlined for better orientiation. During bursoscopy, the constant supply of fluid into the subacromial space leads to a edematous swelling of tissue which impedes exact orientation on the body surface.

- Cushing cannula. This cannula produces a higher outflow. Especially when the view is obstructed by bleeding into the subacromial space, an increased exchange of fluid can enhance vision. The cannula is not used to increase the inflow, since this is ensured by a fluid bag with a thick outflow cannula (5 mm), attached to the ceiling (see Chap. 3).
- Injection needles. These facilitate orientation as they are used to delineate the anterior rim of the acromion, the AC-joint and the coracoacromial ligament.
- Electrosurgical knife. Instead of using expensive standard electrosurgical knives, we use an especially manufactured diathermic tip with a length of 10 cm in our clinic. This needlelike instrument, which is isolated except for the foremost part of the right-angled tip, is connected to the electrocautery. By varying the current, the cutting device can be used most efficiently. When performing a subacromial decompression, this instrument is not only used to maintain hemostasis but also to dissect the coracoacromial ligament as well as to detach the periosteum from the undersurface of the acromion.
  Note: When using a diathermy, sugar solutions must be used instead of electrolyte solutions.

These instruments are not all that is required for therapeutic interventions in the subacromial space (e.g., arthroscopic acromioplasty); supplementary instruments, some of which are especially manufactured, are necessary (see Chap. 7).

Positioning

A detailed explanation of the positioning of the patient for arthroscopy is given in Chap. 3. The same position is used for bursoscopy. In the lateral position the traction weight is increased by 1–2 kg to ensure better extension of the arm. When using the "beach-chair position" this is not necessary, as the action of gravity on the arm increases the longitudinal traction distally. The elbow brace remains unchanged as the easily controllable external and internal rotatory movements of the upper arm are very helpful for orientation in the bursal space.

Portals

• Posterior portal (portal for the arthroscope). For both bursoscopy and arthroscopy, the sheath is introduced through the posterior portal 1 cm distal and 1.5 cm medial to the acromial angle.

The portals for the instruments, however, differ from those used in arthroscopy.

• Lateral portal (portal for instrumentation). The skin incision is made approximately 2 cm lateral to the anterior end of the acromion. This is the portal for nearly all the instruments, as most of the subacromial space can be reached.

The structures lying in the bursa can be readily palpated with the probe when the humeral head is rotated externally and internally. Furthermore, small bleeding vessels can be coagulated, the coracoacromial ligament dissected during arthroscopic subacromial decompression, and calcareous deposits removed through this portal. The shaver and the rongeur are also inserted via this portal when performing a debridement.

• Anterior portal (portal for the file). This is situated 1 cm anterior to the lateral midpoint of the acromion. For a purely diagnostic bursoscopy this portal is not necessary. It is mainly used to insert the reciprocating file when performing a subacromial decompression.

All incisions should be made in a longitudinal direction as this corresponds with the tension lines of the skin and thereby reduces the formation of scars and gives a better cosmetic result.

Technical procedure

As previously mentioned, a bursoscopy should always be preceded by an arthroscopy of the glenohumeral joint.

Control of bleeding can be facilitated by taking certain preoperative measures. Possibilities include:

1. Increasing pressure in the subacromial space:
- by increasing the inflow with a high flow sheath (6.5 mm) or an additional inflow cannula, inserted through a posterior portal
- by using a pressure or volume controlled pump
- by using a pressure cuff which surrounds the fluid bag
- by increasing the water column by hanging the fluid bag as high as possible above the level of the patient.

2. Reduction of systemic blood pressure: certainly the most effective method but only possible under general anesthesia. The mean arterial blood pressure should be 80 mm Hg or the systolic pressure 100 mm Hg.

3. Local vasoconstriction: 2 ml POR 8 (ornithine-vasopressin) diluted to 20 ml are injected into the subacromial space.

On completion of the arthroscopy, the ordinary sheath is exchanged for the special high-flow sheath and advanced under the acromion into the bursa. The index finger of the free hand lies directly anterior to the end of the acromion. The end of the blunt trocar should be palpated.

When the inner layer of the bursa is perforated, the sheath "gives way" indicating that the tip of the trocar has reached the delicate bursal tissue. Medial and lateral movements with the trocar may, on the one hand, remove some of the septae, which hang in front of the arthroscope and obstruct the view into the subacromial space, but, on the other hand, smaller vessels may be damaged and start bleeding, which again leads to a deterioration in vision.

For this reason the scope is inserted first, and only when the view is obstructed by net-like connective tissue is the sheath moved back and forth.

Normal procedure

After having tried pressure cuffs as well as pumps, we have returned to hanging the fluid bag as high as possible. A 10 l container of sugar solution (Resectal) is attached to the ceiling of the operating theater via a pulley. A large bore, high-flow supply system (5 mm outflow cannula, 6.5 mm high-flow sheath) ensures an increased inflow.

A probe is inserted through the lateral incision. Individual septae which obstruct the view are pushed aside. Sometimes these strands of connective tissue cannot be pushed out of the way with the probe, then bursal shaving becomes necessary.

Once satisfactory vision is achieved, the probe is again inserted. With slow internal and external rotation of the forearm, which is bent at an right angle, almost the whole acromial surface of the rotator cuff can be visualized.

The bursa is evaluated up to its arch-like boundary (Figs. 69 and 70). The surface of the tendon is palpated with the probe in order to diagnose any structural irregularity (Fig. 71). Larger, intratendinous calcareous deposits which protrude under the surface of the rotator cuff can easily be located (Fig. 72).

Incomplete as well as complete tendon ruptures situated on the acromial side are detected using the probe and their extent determined (Figs. 73 and 74).

For a better view of the anterior and/or antero-superior parts, the sheath is rotated 180°.

The coracoacromial ligament, coming from a inferomedial direction and running in a supero-lateral direction, serves as a guiding structure. This ligament is located and followed to its insertion on the undersurface of the acromion (Fig. 75).

When an impingement syndrome is present, slow internal and external rotation of the upper arm, with the traction weight temporarily removed, leads to a constriction of the subacromial space in certain places because the rotator cuff is brought close to the inferior acromial surface [5]. Upon the completion of an arthroscopic subacromial decompression, the extent of the acromioplasty can be determined by the increase in space [3; J Esch, pers. comm.].

Percutaneously inserted needles delineate the width of the coracoacromial ligament and can be used as landmarks (Fig. 76).

A detailed inspection and/or palpation of the underside of the humeral fornix completes the diagnostic bursoscopy. The acromio-clavicular joint may be identified by the yellowish fatty tissue which is often found on its undersurface or by the motions produced when repeated pressure is applied externally on the lateral clavicule by the examiner's thumb.

References

1. Bigliani LU, Morrison DS, April EW (1986) The morphology of the acromion and its relationship to rotator cuff tears. Orthop Trans 10:216
2. Crass JR, Craig EV, Bretzke C, Feinberg SB (1985) Ultrasonography of the rotator cuff. Radiographics 5:941–953
3. Ellman H (1987) Arthroscopic subacromial decompression: analysis of one- to three-year results. Arthroscopy 3:173–181
4. Hempfling H (1987) Farbatlas der Arthroskopie großer Gelenke. G Fischer, Stuttgart
5. Matthews LS, Fadale PD (1989) Subacromial anatomy for the arthroscopist. Arthroscopy 5:36–40
6. Morrison DS, Bigliani LU (1987) Roentgenographic analysis of the acromial morphology and its relationship to the rotator cuff tears. Orthop Trans 11:439
7. Neer CS (1972) Anterior acromioplasty for the chronic impingement syndrome in the shoulder: a preliminary report. J Bone Joint Surg [Am] 54:41–50
8. Neer CS, Craig EV, Fukuda H (1983) Cuff-tear arthropathy. J Bone Joint Surg [Am] 65:1232–1244
9. Pattee GA, Snyder SJ (1988) Sonographic evaluation of the rotator cuff: correlation with arthroscopy. Arthroscopy 4:15–20
10. Paulos LE, Franklin IL (1990) Arthroscopic shoulder decompression development and application. A five year experience. Am J Sports Med 18:235–244
11. Rapf C, Furtschegger A, Resch H (1986) Die Sonographie als neues diagnostisches Verfahren zur Abklärung von Schulterbeschwerden. Fortschr Geb Röntgenstr Nuklearmed 145:245–264
12. Sperner G, Resch H (1988) Diagnostik des Schultergelenkes – Klinische Untersuchung. In: Resch H, Beck E (eds) Praktische Chirurgie des Schultergelenkes. Frohnweiler, Innsbruck
13. Snyder SJ, Karzel RP, DelPizzo W, Ferkel RD, Friedman MJ (1990) S.L.A.P. lesions of the shoulder. Arthroscopy 6:274–279

6 Arthroscopic Bankart refixation techniques

6.1 Arthroscopic Bankart suture repair

W. Glötzer, H. Resch, and H. Thöni

There is no doubt that arthroscopy has an important role in the diagnosis of recurrent shoulder subluxation [6, 9, 12]. Consequently, a variety of arthroscopic methods have emerged in the treatment of recurrent shoulder subluxation and subsequently that of recurrent dislocation. Johnson published a stapling technique [19], but this has a relatively high complication rate [18, 21]. In this hospital, we have developed a successful extraarticular screw fixation technique (see Chap. 6.3). Morgan published a suturing technique which originally entailed tying the sutures posteriorly and, in the latest modification, anteriorly over the glenoid labrum [22]. A similar technique was described by Caspari in 1988 [11]. The following suturing technique was published for the first time in 1987 [15]. By using this suturing technique, the Bankart operation in the modification of Bunnell [10] is performed arthroscopically.

Prerequisites for the arthroscopic Bankart suture repair

- Basically normal appearance of the glenoid in multiple roentgenographic views or computed tomography [24, 25],
- no fractures,
- the labrum should be preserved in shape and continuity,
- the lesion must be located in the antero-inferior or antero-superior region of the glenoid rim (not in the region of the superior glenoid pole, i.e., no S.L.A.P. lesion; see Chaps. 6.3 and 6.4).

Indications for Bankart suture repair: are (1) recurrent anterior subluxations and dislocations; (2) detachment of the glenoid labrum in the antero-superior aspect of the glenoid combined with the symptoms of an impingement syndrome (secondary impingement [5, 23]).

Secondary impingement

In our own patient population we repeatedly found complete detachment of the glenoid labrum from the antero-superior aspect of the glenoid in association with impingement syndrome. Commonly, local synovitis with increased vascularization of the capsule between the origin of the long biceps tendon and the antero-superior glenoid rim was an expression of abnormal stress exerted on the capsule secondary to upward migration of the humeral head. Often the biceps tendon and the glenoid labrum were also included in the synovial injection. When the labrum was well preserved, its reattachment led to a significant improvement of the impingement symptoms. However, refixation is only useful when the labrum is largely preserved in shape and continuity. If it is already rather damaged, arthroscopic subacromial decompression (ASD) is the preferred treatment (see also Chaps. 4 and 5). This type of impingement syndrome, secondary in occurrence, should be distinguished from primary impingement syndrome, which arises from the roof of the shoulder [23].

Particular instrumentation

The suturing set (Storz, Acufex) (Fig. 77) consists of a sheath with two cannulas with connected lumina. The cannula centers are 4 mm (Storz) or 5 mm (Acufex) apart and the end is formed into a step (Storz), measuring 3 mm. More recently we prefer a double-lumen cannula with an oblique end (Acufex), because this allows the introduction of the cannula without a trocar sheath. So-called Bankart needles are used, as well as a pointed and a blunt trocar. Absorbable suture material with a thickness of 0 and/or 1 is also used.

Suturing technique

Anesthesia

Either regional or general anesthesia are possible. When using regional anesthesia (interscalene block), the antero-inferior shoulder region (T1 and 2) may sometimes not be completely anesthetized (see Chap. 2). However, this is a rare occurrence and only of significance when using the antero-inferior portal.

Positioning and draping

There are, in principle, two positions.

(1) Lateral recumbent position.   The patient is placed in the lateral recumbent position with the upper part of the body inclined 30° posteriorly (see Chap. 3). Posterior inclination positions the plane of the socket in a nearly horizontal plane, which greatly facilitates orientation. The shoulder blade must be freely accessible. Traction is achieved through an elbow support with the arm in a right-angled position to enable the rotation of the humeral head (arthroscopic elbow brace; Gell, Innsbruck; see Chap. 3). The upper arm is abducted 30 to 40°. Further abduction is not recommended because of the possible injury to the musculocutaneous nerve when advancing towards the inferior portion of the glenoid rim. The traction weight is 4 kg (women) and 5 kg (men). A tightly rolled cloth is placed in the axilla and serves as a fulcrum for distension of the joint.

(2) Half-sitting position.   Lately we have come to prefer the half-sitting position (beach-chair position [1, 27]) instead of the lateral recumbent position (see Chap. 3). The patient is

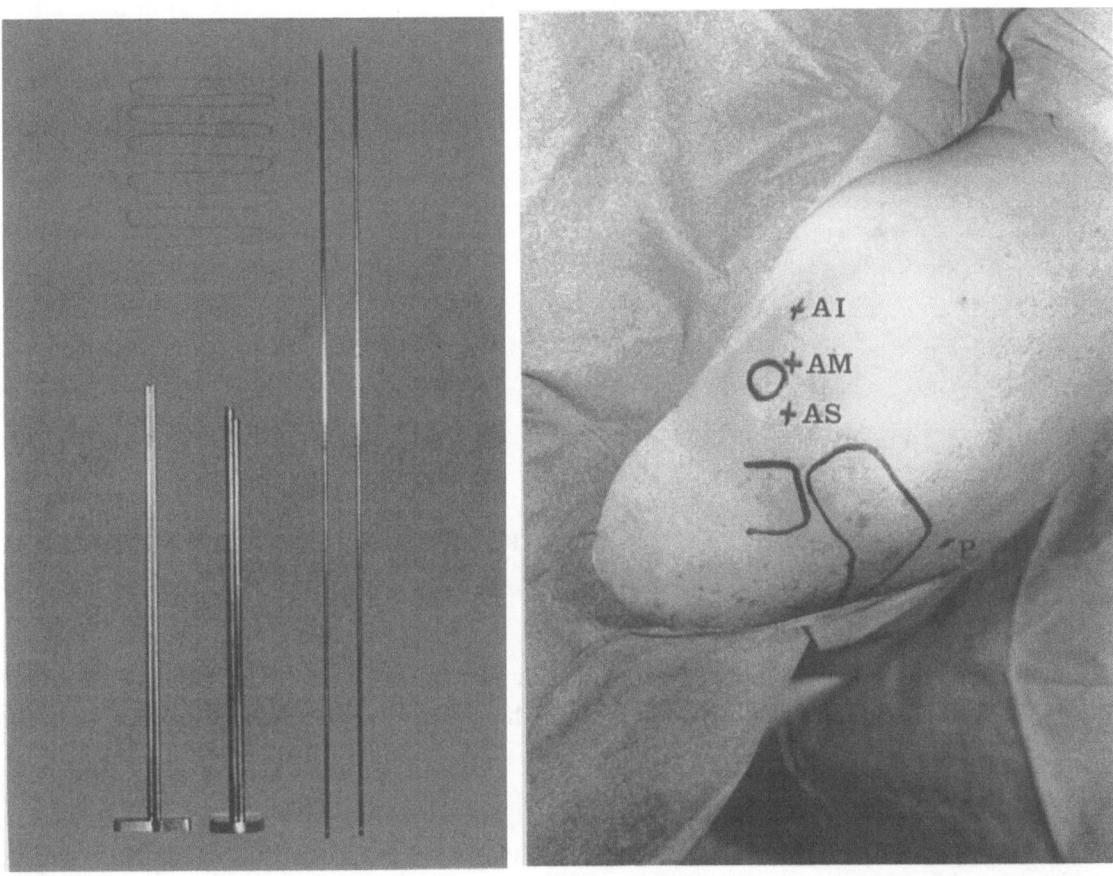

Fig. 77   Fig. 78

Fig. 77. Instrumentation: blunt trocars, double-lumen cannula, Bankart needles, suture material (size 1)

Fig. 78. Right shoulder joint with landmarks and portals (cranial view). *P* Posterior portal (scope), *AS* antero-superior portal, *AM* anterior middle portal, *AI* antero-inferior portal

seated on a cushion level with the edge of the table with the effect that the whole shoulder blade is positioned lateral to and above the edge of the operating table. (Note: When using this technique the whole shoulder blade must be freely accessible!) The patient's head is supported by a head rest. The upper part of the body is stabilized by a lateral support. The arm of the patient is placed in the arthroscopic elbow brace with a traction weight of 2–3 kg. The arm is in 30–40° of abduction. A tightly rolled cloth, 10–15 cm thick, is placed in the axilla to help distract the joint. One advantage of this position is that an unhindered change from arthroscopic to open surgery is possible (as long as the swelling of the shoulder is not too extensive). Furthermore, the patients consider this position comfortable (under regional anesthesia) and the upper part of the body does not get wet. To date, there have been no major drawbacks. The camera must nevertheless be protected from water flowing off the

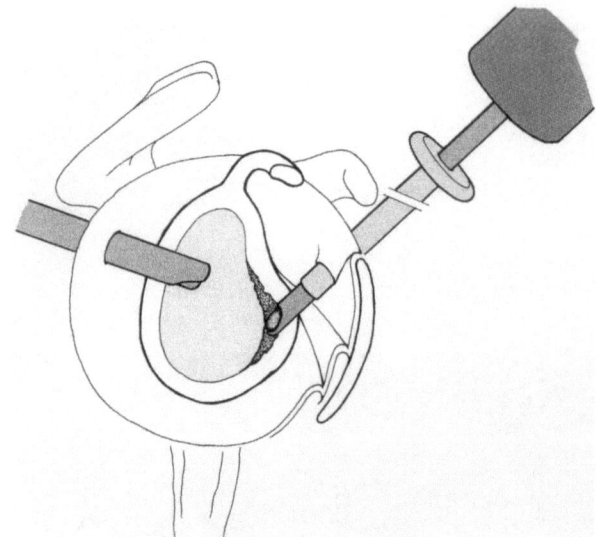

Fig. 79. Abrasion of glenoid rim with ball-tip burr

sheath as the picture will otherwise be blurred. For this purpose we use a rubber diaphragm, which is taken from a disposable cannula (Acufex), and which is slipped onto the sheath [1].

Portals

The landmarks and portals are outlined prior to the operation. We differentiate between the posterior portal for the scope, which is placed 1.5 cm medial and 1 cm inferior to the acromial angle, and three anterior portals (Fig. 78).

●   The anterior middle portal (standard portal) is placed directly lateral to the coracoid tip. This portal is used to insert the double-lumen cannula when performing an intraarticular suture repair. For accurate anterior portal placement the Wissinger rod can be used. First, the scope is advanced to the site of perforation in the joint at the superior margin of the tendon of the subscapularis muscle. The scope is replaced by the Wissinger rod which is then advanced through the sheath to just under the skin. A skin incision is made where a bulging can be seen. The 4 mm guiding trocar and the 7 mm cannula for the instruments are slid over the end of the Wissinger rod. The plastic cannula is inserted into the joint over the Wissinger rod with a rotatory motion. The rod is removed and the scope is again inserted into the sheath.

●   Another anterior portal is the antero-inferior portal which is placed 1.5 to 2 cm inferior to the standard portal and is used for the introduction of the double-lumen cannula when performing the extraarticular suturing technique (mind the musculocutaneous nerve; see also Chap. 6.3).

●   Finally, there is the antero-superior portal which is placed 1 cm superior to the standard portal. This portal is only used when two instruments have to be inserted simultaneously using an anterior approach (e.g., double-lumen cannula via antero-inferior portal and probe

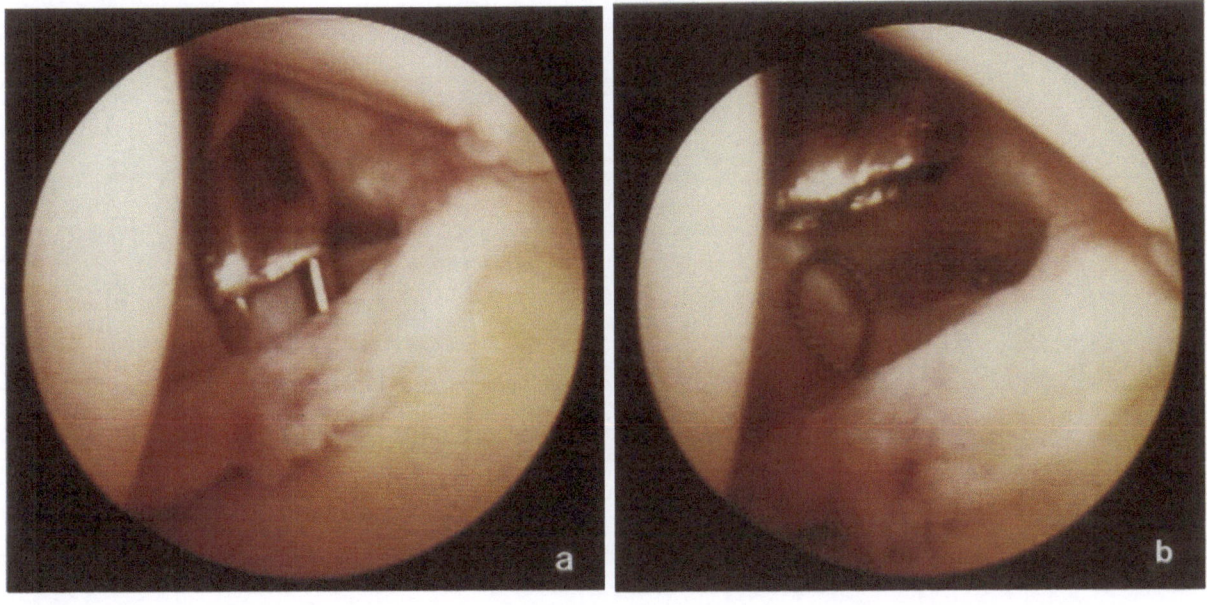

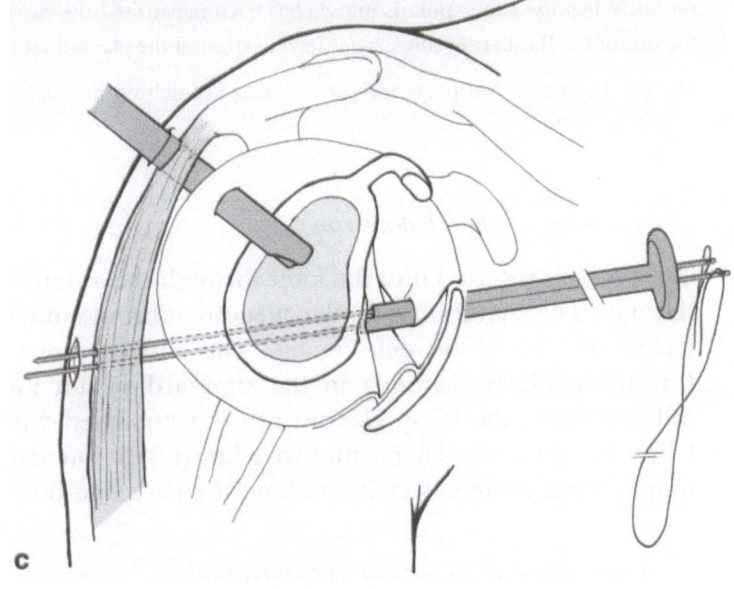

Fig. 80. Intraarticular suturing technique. **a** Detached labrum of the antero-superior aspect of the glenoid speared by the Bankart needles; (double-lumen cannula with an oblique shaped end). **b** U-suture before tightening. **c** Drawing of suturing repair of a Bankart lesion

through antero-superior portal). The distance between the two instruments is thus increased, which facilitates manoeuvring.

The antero-superior portal is also very useful for the introduction of the scope from an anterior direction, e.g., for the precise evaluation of a Bankart lesion. The scope is placed in the plastic cannula, inserted through the antero-superior portal, and introduced into the joint. The anterior glenoid rim can be directly evaluated and the capsule at the scapular neck visualized.

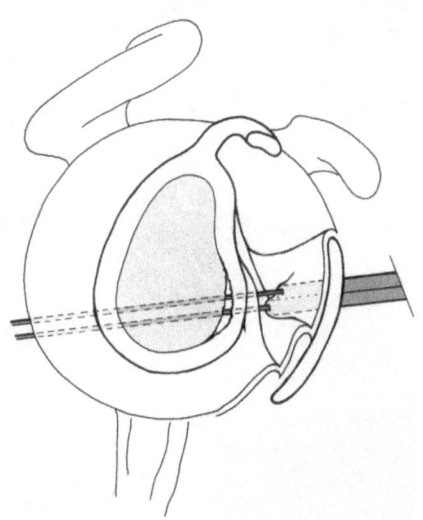

Fig. 81

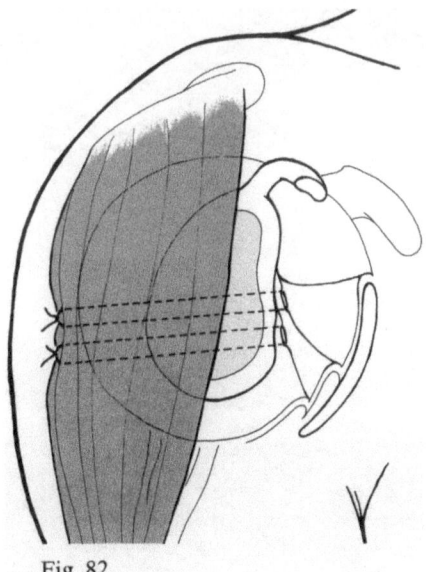

Fig. 82

Fig. 81. Extraarticular (=extracapsular) suturing technique; double-lumen cannula inserted via antero-inferior portal. When the subscapularis muscle has been penetrated the capsule is bulged into the joint and perforated by the tips of the Bankart needles. After having speared the glenoid labrum the needles are driven through the glenoid

Fig. 82. U-sutures tied posteriorly over surface of deltoid muscle

Abrasion of the glenoid rim

The probe is inserted into the joint through the anterior middle portal to palpate the glenoid labrum. The suitability of the glenoid labrum and/or the glenoid rim for the suturing technique should be determined. The shoulder elevator (Acufex) is gradually inserted through a plastic cannula in the standard portal and the dislocated labrum mobilized. Subsequently, the bony glenoid rim is roughened with a Bankart rasp (Acufex) (see also Chap. 6.3, Fig. 94). Then a motorized burr (4.5 mm arthroplasty burr) is inserted and a small longitudinal groove is created along the cartilage-bone junction (Fig. 79).

Intraarticular procedure (Fig. 80)

This technique is used when the detached glenoid labrum is preserved in shape and continuity to such an extent that it can be used for the refixation of the capsule. The double-lumen cannula is inserted via a trocar sheath into the joint through the anterior standard portal (anterior middle portal). The glenoid labrum is speared with a Bankart needle under vision, repositioned on the glenoid rim and tensed in a superior direction. The drill is used to drive the pin inwards in the region of the abraded glenoid rim, parallel to the joint surface, until it can be felt at the back of the shoulder. In the parallel cannula another Bankart needle is inserted under vision, the labrum is perforated and driven through posteriorly parallel to the

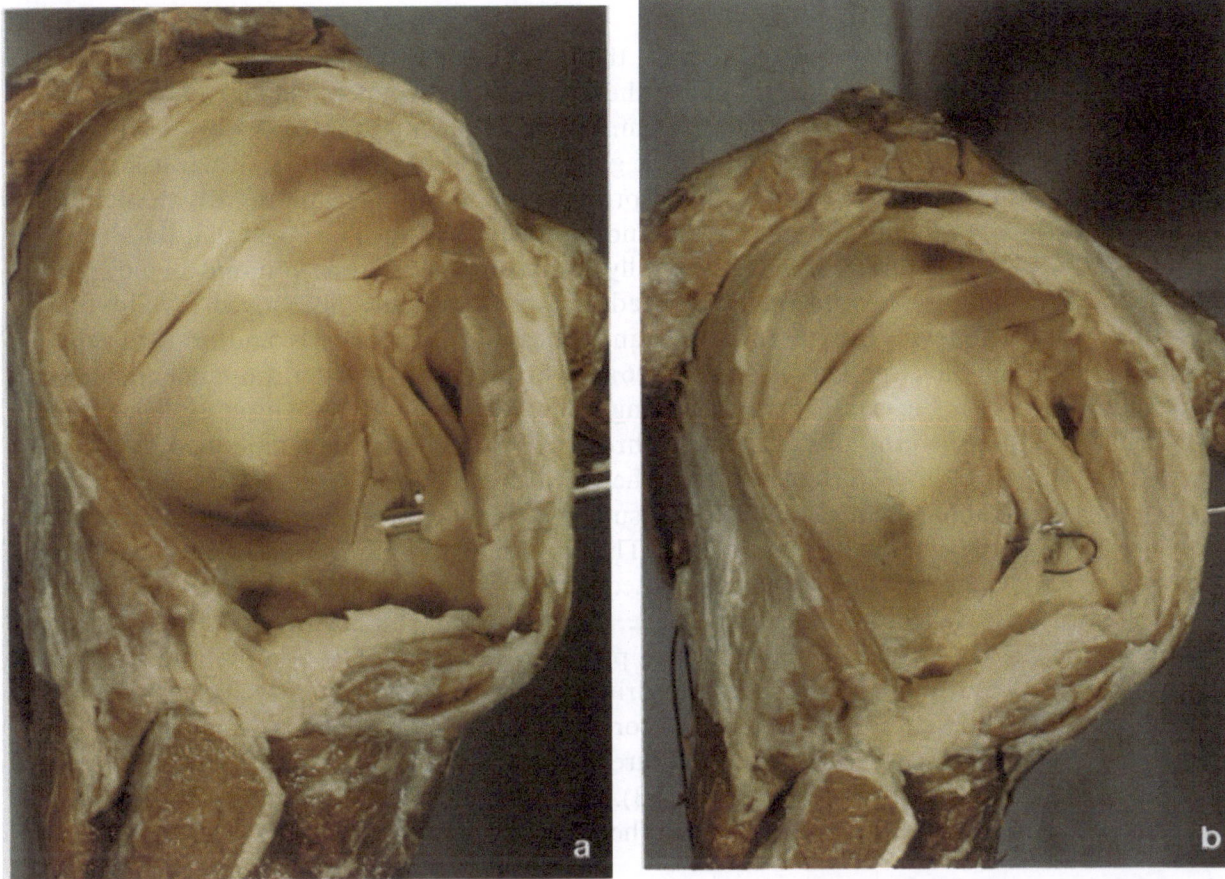

Fig. 83. Anatomical specimen. **a** Double-lumen cannula inserted via antero-inferior portal. **b** U-suture applied; sutures delivered posteriorly through the glenoid

first Bankart needle. A skin incision is made over the tips of the pins. A strand of absorbable suture material, size 1, is threaded through the eyes of the needles. Care must be taken to leave a long enough loop so that the drill wires can be pulled through. Both needles are delivered posteriorly with a grasping forceps. The location of the suture is checked with a probe. The distance between the sutures is 4 mm using a Storz cannula or 5 mm using an Acufex cannula. Whilst tensing the suture tails exiting posteriorly, the arm is rotated externally 30° (via the elbow brace) and the location of the suture and labrum is examined. If the capsule remains slack in this arm position, the origin of the inferior glenohumeral ligament has to be included in the fixation with an additional suture. Depending on the extent of the Bankart lesion, a varied number of sutures (usually 2–3) is applied in the same way.

Extraarticular procedure (Fig. 81)

This technique has been applied only during the last two years. In the case of an extensive anterior detachment with capsular laxity, the inferior glenohumeral ligament has to be reattached in addition to the detached labrum. Through the antero-inferior portal (Fig. 78) the double-lumen cannula is advanced to the glenoid rim, using an extraarticular approach (through a trocar sheath). More recently we prefer a double-lumen cannula with an oblique end (Acufex), because then a trocar sheath is not needed. Care must be taken that the sheath with the trocar is first directed slightly laterally and advanced past the conjoined tendon of the coracobrachial muscle and the short head of the biceps and only moved towards the glenoid rim after having met a hard resistance (head of the humerus and/or tendon of subscapularis muscle) (see Chap. 6.3, Fig. 96a). This ensures that the musculocutaneous nerve is avoided. As the extraarticular suturing technique can produce an excessive block to external rotation, the arm, placed in the arthroscopic elbow brace, is maintained in 30° of external rotation by the assistant surgeon (the forearm shows the degree of rotation).

Using the double-lumen cannula the capsule and/or the labrum is caused to bulge into the joint. This can be observed by the scope. The labrum is speared by the tip of the Bankart needle, repositioned onto the glenoid rim, tensed in a superior-medial direction and the needle driven inwards, parallel to the glenoid surface, until it can be felt posteriorly under the skin. Another needle is inserted over the shorter portion of the suturing cannula and used to perforate the capsule. The second needle is driven through posteriorly as well. After having made certain that the suture has been placed correctly, the traction weight is decreased and the arm brought into internal rotation. The suture tails are tied subcutaneously, strictly epifascially over the deltoid muscle (Figs. 82 and 83). An intraarticular drain is placed through the arthroscopic sheath and left for 12 hours. The incisions are closed with skin sutures.

Postoperative management

Postoperatively, the arm is immobilized in a light shoulder bandage (see Chap. 6.3, Fig. 101) for three to four weeks. A rehabilitation program under the direction of a physical therapist is then begun with external rotation not beyond neutral and flexion not beyond 90°. Full mobilization is started in the sixth postoperative week. At this point the patient is advised to start swimming.

Advantages and drawbacks of the described suture repair technique in comparison to the other techniques described

Simple and relatively quick technique. No metal implant in the joint.

Postoperative immobilization of at least three weeks is required as the knot is located epifascially on the deltoid muscle.

Marked edema of the soft tissue may lead to loosening of the sutures after the swelling has receded, therefore the sutures should be tied as far down as possible.

An already applied suture may be damaged by the needle for the next suture passage. Therefore it is important to place the sutures correctly from the start.

Hazards

(1) Musculocutaneous nerve.   When entering the joint too far medially through the antero-inferior portal, this nerve may be damaged. The antero-inferior portal should not be placed more than 2 cm inferior to the coracoid tip and not further medial than its outer margin. When introducing the cannula with the blunt trocar, it first has to be directed slightly laterally and only turned towards the glenoid rim in a postero-medial direction once a hard resistance (humeral head) is met (Fig. 96 a). Thus the musculocutaneous nerve is safely avoided. Damage of this nerve has never been recorded in our own patients (see also Chap. 6.3).

(2) Suprascapularis nerve.   When driving the needles through posteriorly, they should be aimed at the lateral inferior portion of the infraspinatus muscle. Transient damage to this nerve has occurred in one of our patients.

Patient information

Due to relatively limited experience when compared to open surgery, the arthroscopic Bankart suture repair has not yet been perfected to the same extent as the open procedure. The patient should be informed that it may become necessary to change to an open technique intraoperatively. Furthermore, he/she must be informed of the possibility of neurological damage (musculocutaneous nerve, suprascapularis nerve).

6.2 Arthroscopic three-point Bankart suture repair

P. Habermeyer and E. Wiedemann

The arthroscopic Bankart suturing technique secures the detached glenoid labrum together with the inferior glenohumeral ligament to the glenoid rim using transglenoid sutures. The most important suturing techniques were developed simultaneously in the U.S. by Caspari [11] and Morgan [22]. The technique described below is a modification of Morgan's Bankart technique.

Operative principle

The operative principle of the arthroscopic labrum suture repair is based on the patho-morphology of the Bankart defect. A Bankart lesion is a lesion at the antero-inferior glenoid rim, ranging from a simple detachment of the glenoid labrum to a bony avulsion. Bankart [8] considered the detachment of the labrum to be the cause of recurrent dislocations since the capsule (including the glenohumeral ligaments) is no longer attached to the anterior glenoid rim. Besides its purely mechanical significance as the site of attachment for the capsule and the glenohumeral ligaments, the glenoid labrum also serves as a valvelike lock sealing the glenoid cavity. In cases of labral detachment, this valve mechanism which normal-ly provides negative pressure has been destroyed [16].

The operative principle of the arthroscopic Bankart suture is based on the anatomically sound refixation of the glenoid labrum together with the glenohumeral ligaments to the anterior glenoid rim. After its arthroscopic fixation to the anterior glenoid rim, the glenoid labrum can again function as the site of attachment for the ligaments and as a "sealing ring".

Advantages

The arthroscopic fixation technique causes only minor tissue trauma and makes it possible to dispense with conventional arthrotomy which affects the region of the proprioceptors.

When comparing this technique with the arthroscopic stapling and screw fixation tech-niques, the suture repair has the advantage that there is no danger of complications caused by implants.

The bursting test shows the suturing technique to be twice as stable as the stapling technique [27].

Another advantage of our Bankart modification is that the knots are placed above the posterior portion of the deltoid muscle, posteriorly the knots rest directly over the bony glenoid neck and anteriorly the knot is placed on the labrum under vision and secured against the anterior glenoid rim.

Disadvantages

One general disadvantage is the difficulty of the technique, which can only be performed by an experienced arthroscopic surgeon. Compared with the open procedure, the costs for the acquisition of expensive arthroscopic equipment, special instrumentation and shoulder holder must be taken into consideration.

Another drawback of the closed procedure is that the repair is restricted to the labrum and the inferior glenohumeral ligament. A pathologically enlarged Weitbrecht's foramen or idiopathic redundant and thin joint capsule cannot be closed and repaired by arthroscopic operation.

Finally, we would remind that an incorrect transglenoid drilling technique may damage the suprascapularis nerve.

Indications

Antero-inferior instabilities after major trauma (initial traumatic shoulder dislocation) and/ or repetitive minor trauma, e.g., in sports (throwing athletes), are suited to arthroscopic suture repair. In this hospital, arthroscopic Bankart suture repair is performed after initial traumatic shoulder dislocation or in case of antero-inferiour subluxations producing clinical signs and symptoms.

As no long-term follow-up results for representative patient populations are available to date, arthroscopic repair based on indications other than those mentioned above should only be performed in centers for arthroscopic shoulder surgery where prospectively randomized studies are under way.

A prerequisite for arthroscopic intervention is that the diagnosis has been established by double- or mono-contrast computed tomography, arthroscopy, or MRI.

Generally, the patient population is in the twenty to forty year age group. As Rockwood and collaborators [26] have demonstrated, traumatic anterior shoulder subluxations do not respond to conservative rehabilitation programs. Hence, in contrast to atraumatic forms of instability, physiotherapy does not improve the stability and is a waste of time for the patient.

Contraindications

Massive defects of the glenoid rim (bony Bankart defect), large Hill-Sachs lesions, combined posterior and inferior instabilities as well as multidirectional shoulder instability are to be considered as contraindications for arthroscopic procedures.

If the entire labrum and ligament complex is noted to be frayed and thinned so that the humeral head continuously dislocates over the anterior glenoid rim during arthroscopy, it is best to change to an open surgical technique in a one- or two-stage procedure.

Patient information

Neither the arthroscopic labrum suture repair nor any of the other arthroscopic refixation techniques of the limbus can yet be considered as a standard procedure. The patient should be informed of this and agree to the alternative of open repair. Besides the general risks, specific complications such as a lesion of the brachial plexus caused by traction, damage to the suprascapularis nerve as well as a possible damage to the axillary nerve and the musculo-cutaneous nerve have to be mentioned.

Anesthesia

In principle, it is possible to perform the intervention under regional anesthesia (interscalene block). Due to the attendant circumstances which are uncomfortable for the patient (traction to the arm, drilling noise, lateral position, possible wetness caused by the irrigation fluid) insufflation anesthesia is recommended. We combine insufflation anesthesia with inter-scalene block as this prolongs postoperative analgesia.

The extent and direction of the instability should again be examined in the anesthetized patient. If the shoulder is completely unstable under anesthesia and dislocates immediately after repositioning, it is already clear at this stage that the anteriorly dislocated head of the humerus will make arthroscopic suture repair more difficult.

Positioning and draping

The operation is performed with the patient in the lateral recumbent position, the upper part of the body is inclined approximately 30° posteriorly. The body is stabilized by lateral supports. Care should be taken not to block the scapula with the support at the back of the patient.

The affected arm is extended by means of an arm support (Arthrex) with the shoulder joint in a standard position, and brought into 45° of abduction and 30° of flexion as well as internal rotation. The extension weight is 5 kg for women and 6 kg for men. To facilitate the access to the joint cavity, the arm is extended vertically by a pulley device attached to the upper arm. Covering up to the upper arm is done with a sterile stockinette (Mölnlycke).

Thus it is possible to move the arm during the arthroscopic intervention in compliance with the proviso for sterility and to allow for necessary changes of the position in the shoulder joint.

As an alternative we have recently been performing the operation with the patient in the half-sitting position which is also used in open surgery. Altcheck et al. [2] were the first to report on this, Resch in Innsbruck and Walch in Lyon have also gained experience with this position. The sitting position is suited for the arthroscopic stabilization as well as for all other diagnostic and operative interventions in the glenohumeral and subacromial region. There are a few advantages of the sitting position: less time is required for positioning and anesthesia and no supplementary equipment such as arm supports needed. The position is more convenient when using insufflation anesthesia and more comfortable for the patient in the waking state with interscalene blocking. If the joint has to be opened, no repositioning or renewed disinfection and covering is required.

Portals

The bony landmarks should be delineated with a marker pencil and the skin contours over the scapular spine, the acromion, the AC joint and the coracoid process marked exactly. Thus the exact placement of the portals is facilitated.

We use the following portals for the arthroscopic Bankart suture repair.

- Posterior portal (portal for scope). The posterior portal is placed in the "soft spot", normally approx. 1.5 cm medial and 1 cm distal to the readily palpable posterior acromial angle.
- Superior portal (Neviaser portal). The point of entry for the superior portal lies superior to the supraspinatus fossa directly at the tip of an angle which is bounded by the lateral end of the clavicle and the AC joint anteriorly, laterally by the acromion and posteriorly by the scapular spine. This portal is normally used for water inflow or as the portal giving access to the supraglenoid tuberosity. Puncturing is carried out at a 45° angle to the longitudinal axis of the body and aims directly at the midpoint of the glenohumeral joint.
- Anterior middle portal (standard portal). It is located slightly lateral to the tip of the coracoid process and enters the middle anterior joint cavity above the tendon of the subscapularis muscle. It is used as the standard portal for instrumentation and allows the 7 mm thick plastic cannula to be inserted safely.
- Antero-superior portal [6]. It is located halfway between the coracoid process and the anterior acromial edge and enters the joint between the long biceps tendon and superior margin of the subscapularis tendon. This portal permits an exact visualization of the anterior glenoid rim and, above all, of the scapular neck. It is also necessary when the arthroscope and the instruments are used simultaneously in an anterior approach.

Operative technique

The principle of this method is a stable "three-point knot" directly above the bony rim of the glenoid socket. All three knots are placed epiglenoidally, the anterior knot intraarticularly over the fixed labrum on the anterior glenoid rim. Thus a stable three-point fixation is achieved.

Diagnostic arthroscopy is performed via the posterior portal. Water inflow is either achieved through the arthroscopic cannula with a pump or through the Neviaser portal.

For the placement of the anterior middle portal (standard portal) we use an inside-out technique with the Wissinger rod. First, the arthroscope is advanced between the superior margin of the subscapularis tendon and inferior margin of the long biceps tendon against the anterior joint capsule, then the arthroscope is replaced by the Wissinger rod which is pressed firmly against the anterior capsular wall. After making a stab incision above its point of protrusion, the Wissinger rod is further advanced through the incision in an anterior direction. Now a 4 mm guiding trocar can be attached to the Wissinger rod from an anterior direction and the instrument cannula (7 mm inner diameter) placed over the trocar. Next, the 4 mm guiding trocar is advanced together with the instrument cannula over the guiding rod into the anterior joint cavity without damaging any intraarticular structures. After removing the Wissinger rod, the arthroscope is again inserted from a posterior direction.

The first step is a diagnostic arthroscopy. The probe is used to examine the stability of the long biceps tendon and the glenoid labrum (Fig. 84). If the glenoid labrum is detached, the probe can be advanced subperiosteally to the "Bankart pocket". Uncertainties in the assessment may make it necessary to remove the arthroscope from the posterior portal and insert it through the antero-superior portal. Using the antero-superior approach, the extent of the Bankart lesion and the detachment of the middle and inferior glenohumeral ligament can be determined exactly. Once the extent of the defect has been established, the arthroscope is again inserted through the posterior portal.

The next step includes a careful abrasion of the anterior glenoid rim as far as the scapular neck (Fig. 85). Any residual adhesions and scars must be removed in order to achieve a sufficiently large abraded area in the glenoid neck. The preparation is the same as that for an open Bankart operation. Abrasion of the anterior glenoid rim is performed with a specially designed rasp (Bankart rasp, Acufex) and motorized ball-shaped abrading shavers. Care should be taken to avoid damage to the labrum. Only adequate debridement guarantees that the labrum and capsule heal back to the anterior bony glenoid rim.

Suturing technique

After inserting a grasping stitcher (Arthrex), the labrum is grasped together with the inferior glenohumeral ligament at its lowest possible point of detachment and both are drawn upwards and positioned anatomically at the bony glenoid rim, approximately in a position between 3 and 4 o'clock (Fig. 86). The labrum is to be grasped at its most inferior point and a shift has to be performed.

The cannulated grasping stitcher allows the simultaneous positioning of the labrum and the introduction of a Kirschner wire. A 1.7 mm Kirschner wire with an eye at the end is inserted into the grasping stitcher. It is now drilled through the reduced labrum, with or without the inferior glenohumeral ligament, It is driven transscapularly in an antero-posterior direction, slightly below the articular surface. The drilling direction of the Kirschner wire is 30° inferior to the transverse axis of the articular surface and about parallel or a maximum of 15° medially inclined to it.

The Kirschner wire perforates the skin in the region of the infraspinatus fossa. The exit through the skin must be placed at least 3 cm below the scapular spine so as not to damage the suprascapular nerve. A drill guide in connection with the cannulated grasping stitcher facilitates the safe placement of the wire in the region of the infraspinatus fossa. To prevent the Kirschner wire from penetrating into the glenoid socket, the glenoid surface is observed through the arthroscope during the entire drilling procedure. Two strands of size 2 absorbable suture (Vicryl) are threaded through the eye of the Kirschner wire and then carefully brought out posteriorly. The sutures are pulled out enough to make long suture tails available anteriorly and posteriorly. After having dilated the posterior skin exit with a clamp, the two posterior suture tails are tied to form a 3–4 mm thick "mulberry knot". The sutures are then drawn retrograde back under the skin until the thick knot is seated at the posterior exit of the drill-channel on the glenoid rim. The sutures are securely fixed if a firm resistance can be felt and the shoulder joint can be pulled forward when applying traction. Thus, the first set of sutures has been placed.

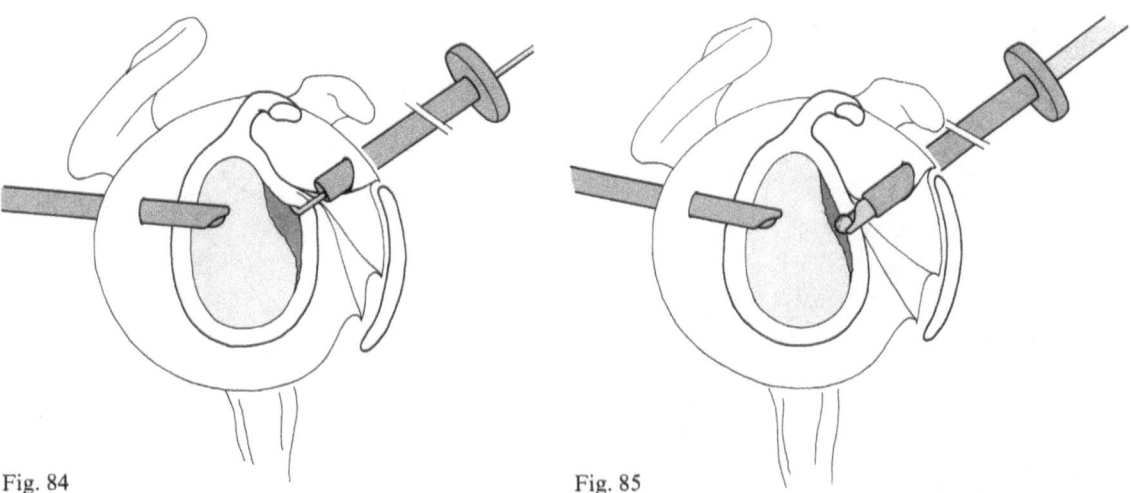

Fig. 84   Fig. 85

Fig. 84. Assessment of the Bankart defect with the probe. Detachment of the glenoid labrum together with the inferior glenohumeral ligament from the anterior glenoid rim

Fig. 85. Abrasion of the anterior glenoid rim with the abrader

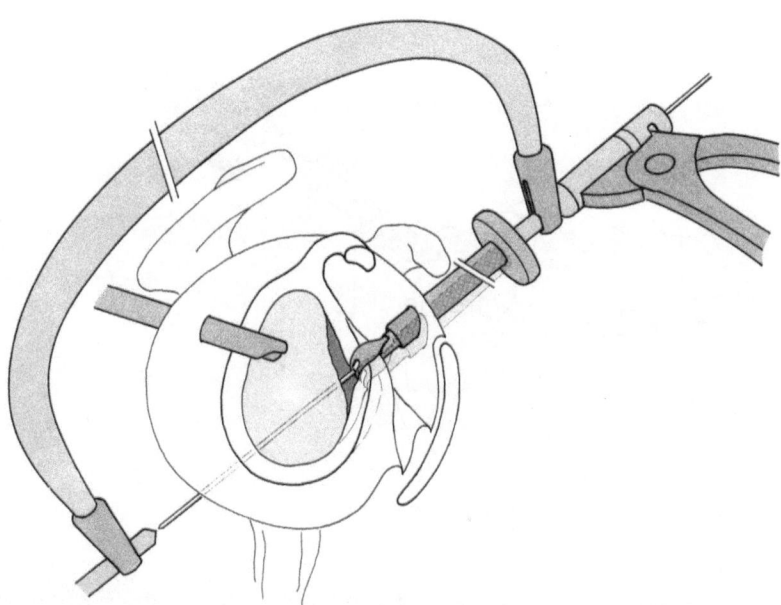

Fig. 86. Transfixation of the glenoid labrum with Kirschner wire (with an eye for the strand). Reduction of the labrum together with the inferior glenohumeral ligament by means of the cannulated grasping stitcher. Use of a drill guide for safe positioning, thus protecting the suprascapularis nerve

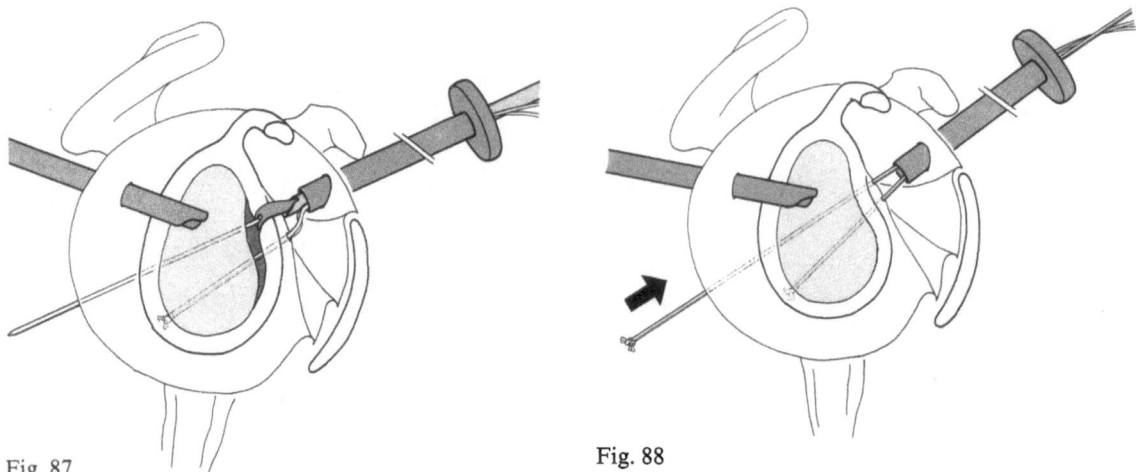

Fig. 87

Fig. 88

Fig. 87. Transfixation of the glenoid labrum with K-wire. Introduction of the second K-wire at 2 o'clock past the first placed set of sutures and transscapular delivery posteriorly

Fig. 88. Firm fixation of the two mulberry knots on the posterior glenoid rim

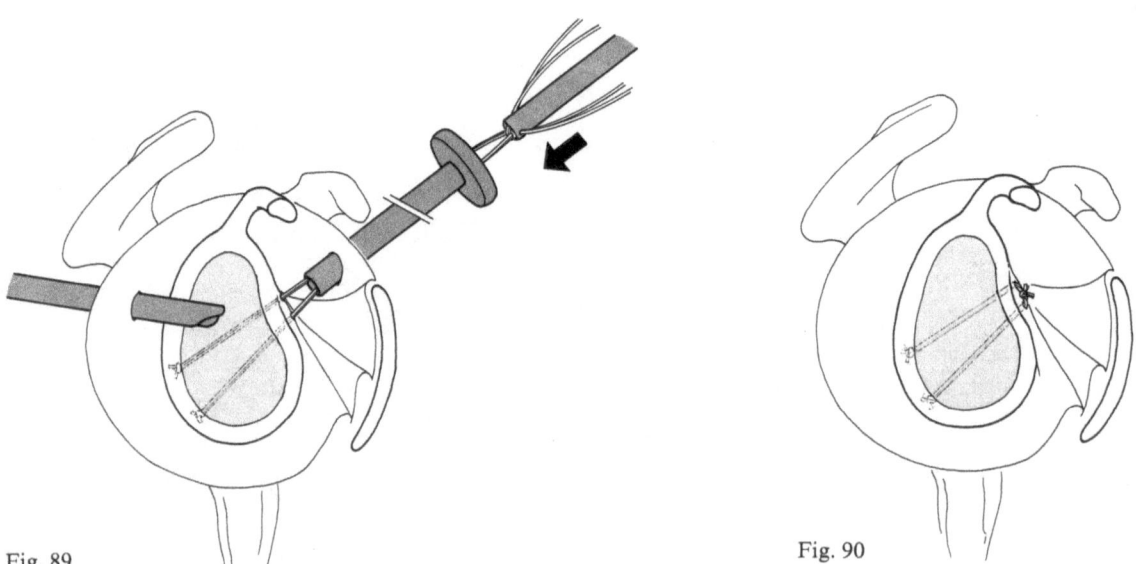

Fig. 89

Fig. 90

Fig. 89. Tying the sutures anteriorly with the knot pusher. The two sets of sutures are tied exteriorly and pushed onto the labrum by means of the knot pusher

Fig. 90. "Three-point knot technique". Completion of the suture over the ligament labral complex with two mulberry knots posteriorly and a double knot anteriorly

We then repeat the same procedure for the placement of a second set of sutures. The cannulated grasping stitcher is again inserted through the plastic cannula past the first set of sutures. In a more superior position (2 o'clock) the stitcher is used to grasp the detached labrum and to resite it correctly onto the anterior glenoid rim. The 1.7 mm thick Kirschner wire is inserted through the instrument and is used to spear the seized labrum and to fix it anatomically back to the anterior joint socket. The drill direction runs at a 15° angle medial to the joint surface and simultaneously at a 15–30° angle to the first Kirschner wire, that is to say, sagittal and horizontal to the joint socket. Next, the second Kirschner wire is drilled through posteriorly. The two exits must be placed in a perpendicular line below the scapular spine, between 3 cm superior and a maximum of 10 cm inferior to it to avoid neurological damage (Fig. 87).

A second set of sutures is now threaded through the eye of the Kirschner wire and delivered posteriorly by means of the wire. We also tie the posterior loose ends of the second set of sutures to themselves several times with a second stable mulberry knot and, after having dilated the drill-channel subcutaneously, pull the suture retrograde under the skin again until the thick knot is seated on the glenoid rim at the exit of the second-channel. Now both mulberry knots are firmly fixed in place on the posterior glenoid rim (Fig. 88).

Subsequently, the two anterior sets of sutures are tied intraarticularly. A knot pusher (Arthrex) allows us to tie the two anterior suture tails over the labrum by placing the knots externally and then pushing them through the instrument cannula with the knot pusher onto the labrum (Fig. 89). As two sets of sutures have been placed, a single knot in each suture set is first advanced anteriorly over the labrum by means of a knot pusher. A single throw or double throw, in the same direction, is made and then pushed firmly to the labrum by means of a knot pusher while applying traction to the two suture tails.

In the case where a single throw was used, a second throw is tied in the same direction, in order to prevent it from being prematurely blocked by the first throw when advancing it.

The procedure is then repeated by using one strand from each suture set. The sutures are then tied repeatedly, alternating suture strands used. All in all, the sutures are tied five times to enture absolute stability of the knot. Thus the "three-point suture technique" is completed; two mulberry knots are placed posteriorly on the glenoid rim, and one large counter knot is placed anteriorly on the glenoid labrum (Fig. 90).

Postoperative management

The arm is immobilized in a Gilchrist bandage for 3 weeks. The subsequent physiotherapy is in keeping with the guidelines established for therapy after open surgery of anterior shoulder instabilities [17].

Defects and hazards

Specific hazards of the transglenoid Bankart technique are damage to the suprascapularis nerve as well as damage to the glenoid surface due to incorrect drilling technique.

Generally, defects are due to an incorrect assessment of the Bankart lesion, especially when the subperiosteal detachment from the anterior glenoid rim and insufficiency of the inferior glenohumeral ligament have not been determined adequately. Failing to notice a habitual component such as a general joint laxity constitutes another error and in this case the insufficiency of the glenohumeral capsule and ligament complex cannot be repaired with the applied technique.

Damage to the axillary nerve, musculocutaneous nerve, and cephalic vein can and should be avoided in all arthroscopic stabilization operations.

"Insufficient postoperative physiotherapy, lacking personal follow-up of the patient" [28] may jeopardize the success of the operation. The physiotherapist in charge of the postoperative treatment must either be informed personally or by a detailed written postoperative treatment plan. Thorough follow-up, counselling and early patient evaluation ensures a successful outcome.

Errors in the postoperative rehabilitation phase are premature external rotation and premature sporting activities (within six months after the operation).

6.3 Arthroscopic screw fixation techniques

H. Resch, K. Golser, and A. Kathrein

The aim of the Bankart procedure is the repair of the so-called "Bankart lesion" located at the antero-inferior glenoid rim [7, 8]. Attempts have been made in the last few years to achieve the same results without opening the soft tissue layer by using an arthroscopic approach [11, 15, 16, 19, 22]. This was attempted using arthroscopically implanted staples, which were inserted intraarticularly to reattach the detached labrum-capsule complex (Bankart lesion) to the bony glenoid rim. However, this technique resulted in a significant incidence of complications such as loosening and breakage of implants [18, 21]. We believe that the reason for the high complication rate was to be found in the unfavorable pull of the capsule on the intraarticularly located staples. A screw fixation technique originally developed for the refixation of labrum detachments at the superior pole of the glenoid (S.L.A.P. lesion [30]) has also proved its worth in cases of recurrent shoulder dislocations or subluxations, and fresh fractures of the glenoid rim. Except for cases of S.L.A.P. lesions, the screw fixation technique differs from the stapling technique insofar as the cannulated screws are placed extraarticularly (extracapsularly) into the glenoid rim with the aid of a guide wire, so that the implant does not lie in the joint. This ensures that the capsule exerts less traction on the screws and consequently the complication rate is lower (Fig. 91 a and b). As with this technique the joint is not entered at the upper margin of the subscapularis tendon, but through the subscapularis muscle. The capsule can be reattached directly in the center of the Bankart lesion. Moreover, a hyperlax capsule can be shortened. Intraarticularly placed screws are only used when the screws cannot be placed extraarticularly, such as when reattaching the labrum in a S.L.A.P. lesion. In order to avoid the necessity of later removal of intra-articularly placed metal screws, we have recently come to use absorbable tacks for the refixation of S.L.A.P. lesions (see Chap. 6.4). The use of screws has also proved appropriate for the arthroscopic refixation of fragments of the glenoid rim.

Indications for the arthroscopic screw fixation technique

- Recurrent shoulder dislocation or subluxation provided that the glenoid is not too small, too flat or tilted too far anteriorly [24] – extraarticular placement of screws.
- Acute fractures of the glenoid rim – extraarticular placement of screws.
- Complete detachment of the glenoid labrum at the origin of the long biceps tendon (S.L.A.P. lesion) – intraarticular placement of screws is obligatory.

The extraarticular screw fixation technique should only be performed with two experienced arthroscopists, one managing the scope and the other placing the screws.

Screw insertion is performed using a specially designed arthroscopic screw fixation system (Leibinger, Mühlheim, Federal Republic of Germany). Cannulated 2.7 mm self-tapping titanium screws are inserted over a guide wire. The screw can be released at any point from a special screw holding device, but also can be grasped again which allows intraarticularly placed screws to be removed arthroscopically (Fig. 92 a–d). (Extraarticularly located screws can only be removed arthroscopically while the guide remains in place.)

Extraarticular Bankart screw fixation technique for recurrent shoulder dislocation

Anesthesia

The arthroscopic Bankart screw fixation can be performed under general anesthesia as well as regional anesthesia (interscalene block).

Positioning and draping

Basically two positions are possible (see Chap. 3): (1) lateral position; (2) half-sitting position. During the past 24 months, arthroscopic interventions in the shoulder have almost exclusively been performed with the patient in a half-sitting position (beach-chair position).

Draping is done with sterile adhesive tissue. The arm, suspended in the arthroscopic elbow brace, is wrapped in a sterile "thigh stocking" (Stockinette large, Mölnlycke). A tightly rolled cloth with a diameter of approximately 10–15 cm is placed in the axilla, it acts as a fulcrum which distracts the humeral head in a lateral direction. The coracoid process and the acromion are outlined with a marking pencil.

Portals

The portals are also outlined preoperatively with a marking pencil. For the extraarticular screw fixation technique the standard anterior portal (anterior middle portal) is not used. However, two additional portals are required (Fig. 93).

- Posterior portal (portal for the scope). Normally this portal lies 1.5 cm medial and 1 cm inferior to the acromial angle.
- Antero-superior portal [6]. This is located about 1 cm superior to the tip of the coracoid. The joint is entered slightly anterior to the long biceps tendon. Because of the superior displacement of this portal, the distance to the antero-inferior portal is increased. This facilitates working when two instruments are needed simultaneously, e.g., for extraarticular Bankart screw fixation or screw fixation of an antero-inferior fragment of the glenoid rim. The probe, inserted through this portal, maintains the fragment in the reduced position, while the cannula with the blunt trocar is introduced via the antero-inferior portal. The antero-superior portal is also very useful for the insertion of the scope to accurately evaluate the Bankart lesion. The scope is slipped into the plastic cannula (Acufex, Arthrex), which is placed in the antero-superior portal, and thus introduced into the joint. The anterior glenoid rim can be evaluated directly and the inferior recesses at the neck of the scapula viewed.

● Antero-inferior portal. This is placed 1.5 to 2 cm inferior to the lateral edge of the coracoid tip. The cannula with the blunt trocar is inserted via this portal through the subscapularis muscle towards the antero-inferior rim of the glenoid. When inserting the trocar sheath, it must first be directed slightly laterally until the conjoint tendon is safely passed. After meeting the humeral head (hard resistance), the cannula is swept postero-medially towards the glenoid rim and advanced through the subscapularis muscle (Fig. 96 a). The change of direction ensures that the musculocutaneous nerve is avoided.

Preparation of the glenoid rim

This is the same as described for the arthroscopic Bankart suture repair, but the instruments are inserted via the antero-superior portal: A plastic cannula (Acufex, Arthrex) is used for the introduction of the instruments. First, the arthroscopic elevator (shoulder elevator; Acufex) is used to mobilize the displaced glenoid labrum and subsequently the bony rim of the glenoid is roughened with an arthroscopic rasp (Bankart rasp; Acufex) (Fig. 94 a and b). Then a small longitutinal groove is performed with the motorized burr (arthroplasty burr 4.5 mm; Concept) (Fig. 95 a and b).

Screw fixation technique

The 6 mm thick trocar sheath with the cannulated blunt trocar (drill guide) is advanced to the glenoid rim via the antero-inferior portal (Fig. 96 a and b). The trocar sheath is first directed slightly laterally and advanced until meeting hard resistance (humeral head) and then redirected posteromedially towards the glenoid rim. The trocar sheath with the blunt trocar is advanced anteriorly through the subscapularis muscle to the joint capsule until the latter protrudes into the joint. The arm is placed in the right-angled elbow brace (see Chap. 3) and rotated externally about 30°. This external rotation prevents the capsule from being shortened too much and places the tendon of the subscapularis muscle lateral to the glenoid rim, which facilitates perforation of the subscapularis muscle by the blunt trocar. A 1 mm

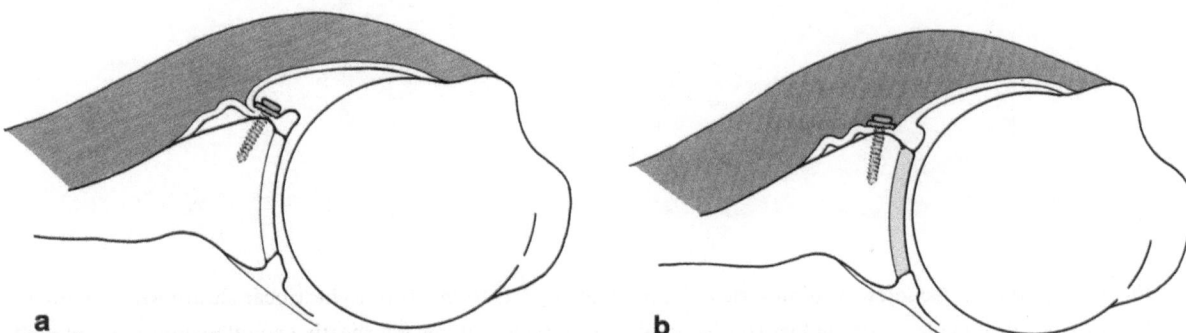

Fig. 91. Intra- and extraarticular placement of screws. **a** Intraarticularly; stress on screw head due to traction of capsule with subsequent loosening of screw. **b** Extraarticularly; tangential stress on screw head due to traction of capsule at external rotation; after healing only traction of capsule at the glenoid rim

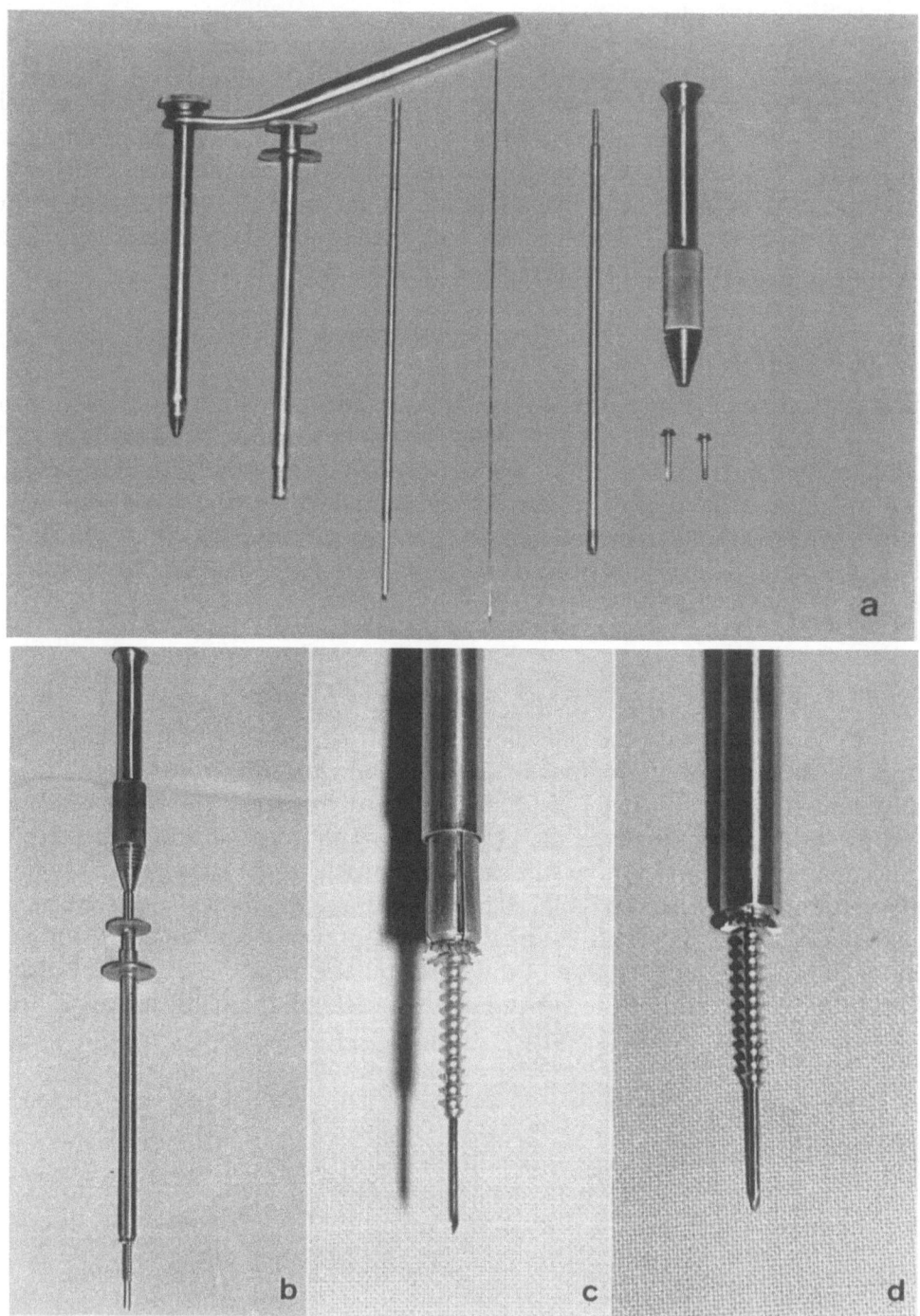

Fig. 92. "Arthroscopic screw fixation system." **a** Individual parts from left to right: trocar sheath with cannulated blunt trocar (drill guide), screw holder consisting of tension plier and tension sheath, cannulated burr, 1 mm guide wire, screw driver, handle, cannulated titanium screws with convex washer. **b** Screw driver with tension pliers, tension sheath, inserted screw and central guide wire. **c** Locking mechanism open; tension sheath retracted, screw inserted loosely into tension plier. **d** Locking mechanism closed; tension sheath pushed forward, screw inserted tightly into tension plier

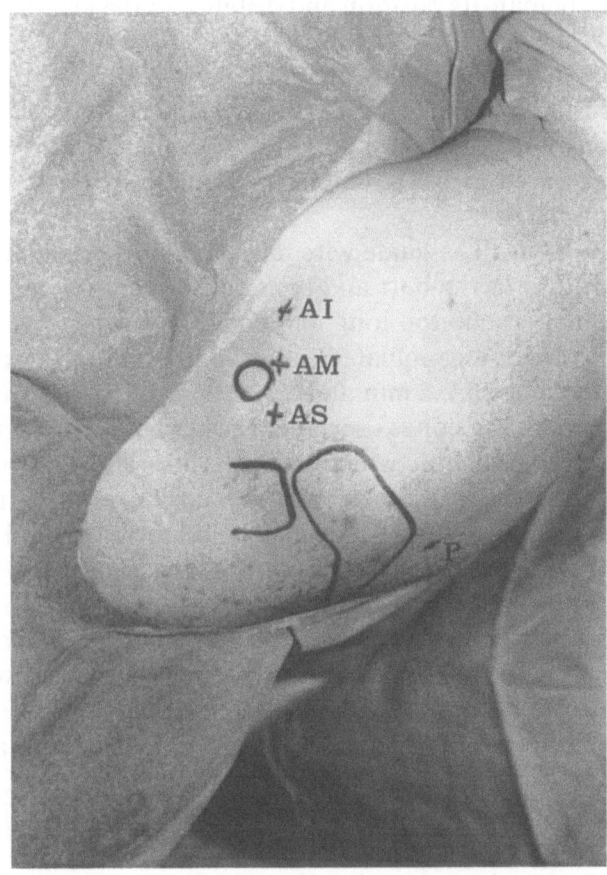

Fig. 93. Portals to shoulder joint (right shoulder, cranial view); one posterior (*P*) portal (scope) and three anterior portals: antero-superior (*AS*), anterior middle (*AM*) and antero-inferior (*AI*) portal

Kirschner wire is advanced through the drill guide until it perforates the glenoid labrum. The speared labrum is reduced to its original site by means of the Kirschner wire, the tip of which should come to rest in the previously drilled groove (Fig. 96 c, e, and f). For easier identification of a suitable site for the insertion of the Kirschner wire, a probe is introduced through the antero-superior portal to lift the glenoid labrum a little near the tip of the wire (Fig. 96 d). At a suitable site on the bony glenoid rim, the Kirschner wire is placed under arthroscopic control and drilled into the glenoid rim and/or scapular neck as far as the opposite cortex (Fig. 96 g). Although the screw is placed completely extracapsularly, the guide wire has to be placed at a distance of at least 3 mm from the free edge of the cartilage because the diameter of the washer is 5 mm. The distance can be easily assessed by using the probe.

Under no circumstances should the wire be positioned in the articular cartilage. Using the probe, which is introduced through the antero-superior portal, the glenoid labrum is kept elevated by the assistant so that all further operative steps such as drilling and tightening the screws until reapproximation of the labrum can be observed through the gap between labrum and glenoid rim. A prerequisite for this is adequate mobilization of the labrum at the start of the operation. If a direct view of the Kirschner wire cannot be achieved, the probe is used to palpate its position and distance to the glenoid rim which should be about 3 mm (= length of the probe).

After removal of the drill guide and shortening of the guide wire slightly above the edge of the trocar sheath (see below), the cannulated 2.2 mm drill is inserted over the guide wire and a drill hole is made (Fig. 97a and b). While drilling, the mark on the sheath should be observed in order to prevent drilling to far which would cause the guide wire to become displaced.

Note: The guide wire must be cut at or slightly above the edge of the trocar sheath after drilling as the burr and the screw driver are only cannulated to a certain point! The wire will otherwise be too long and could be bent.

Next, a cannulated self-tapping titanium screw with an outer diameter of 2.7 mm, inner diameter of 2.2 mm and a length of 16 to 18 mm is placed in the screw holding device. The screw has a convex serrated washer with a diameter of 5 mm which rotates freely around the screw neck but which cannot slide off. The screw, together with the screw holder and cannulated screw driver, is advanced over the wire to the glenoid rim and tightened until the washer firmly presses the glenoid labrum with the adherent joint capsule to the glenoid rim (Fig. 98a–d). The procedure of pressing can be closely observed through the scope. The probe is used to check the refixation of the capsule and the cartilage is inspected with the scope to make sure no metal is seen shining through. Also, the arm is externally rotated to check the correct length of the reattached capsule. External rotation up to 30° should be possible. Subsequently, the screw driver and the screw holding device with the guide wire are removed. Depending on the extent of the Bankart lesion, a second screw is inserted in the same manner 1 cm from the first. The location of the second screw has to be anticipated prior to placement of the first screw (Fig. 99a and b).

Extraarticular removal of screws.   This is only possible arthroscopically prior to removing the guide wire. Therefore the reattached joint capsule and the joint cartilage must be carefully examined before removing the guide wire. The screw driver is advanced to the screw over the guide wire and the screw is loosened a few threads. The screw holder, consisting of tension plier and tension sheath, is advanced along the shaft of the screw driver over the head of the screw. By means of the tension sheath, the head of the screw is firmly fixed in the tension plier (Fig. 92c and d). The screw can then be easily removed.

Hazards

(1) Musculocutaneous nerve.   If the blunt trocar is inserted through the antero-inferior portal too medially and inferiorly (extraarticular screw fixation) this nerve may be damaged. Although a nerve usually evades a blunt instrument, it should not be introduced further medially than the outer margin of the coracoid tip and not further inferiorly than 2 cm when using the antero-inferior portal. The introduction of the trocar has to be performed as described above (Fig. 96a).

(2) Screw loosening.   This only constitutes a problem when the screws are located intraarticularly. Screw loosening has not occurred in any case operated on by the extraarticular technique so far.

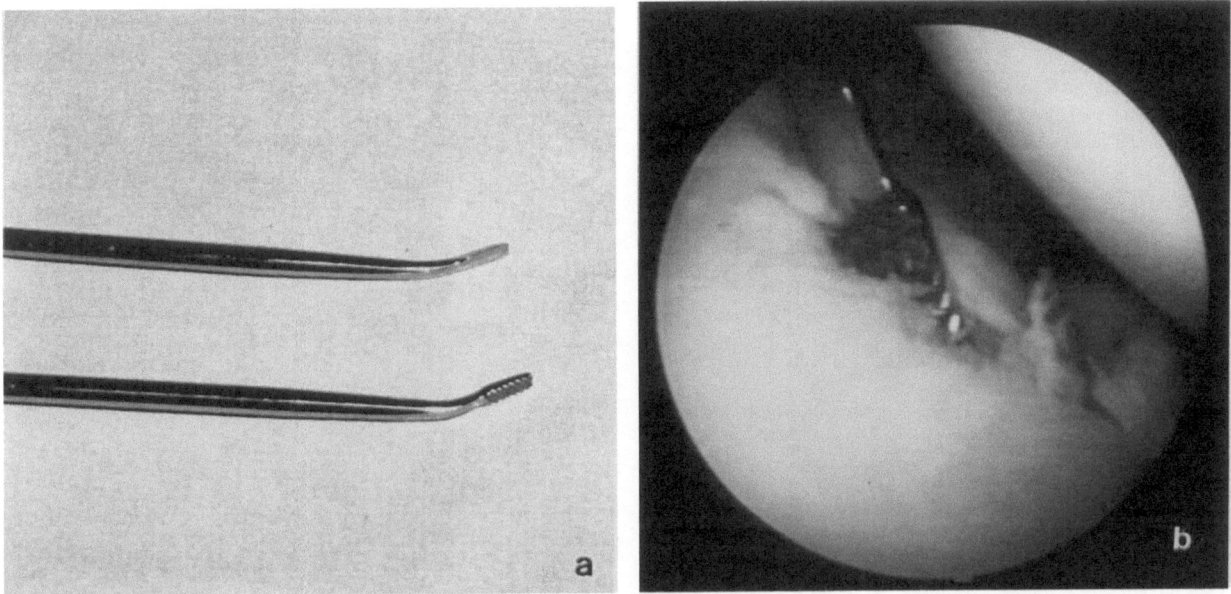

Fig. 94. Instrumentation for abrasion of the glenoid rim. **a** Shoulder elevator (above) for mobilization of the labrum and Bankart rasp (below) for roughening of glenoid rim. **b** Arthroscopic view. Roughening with Bankart rasp

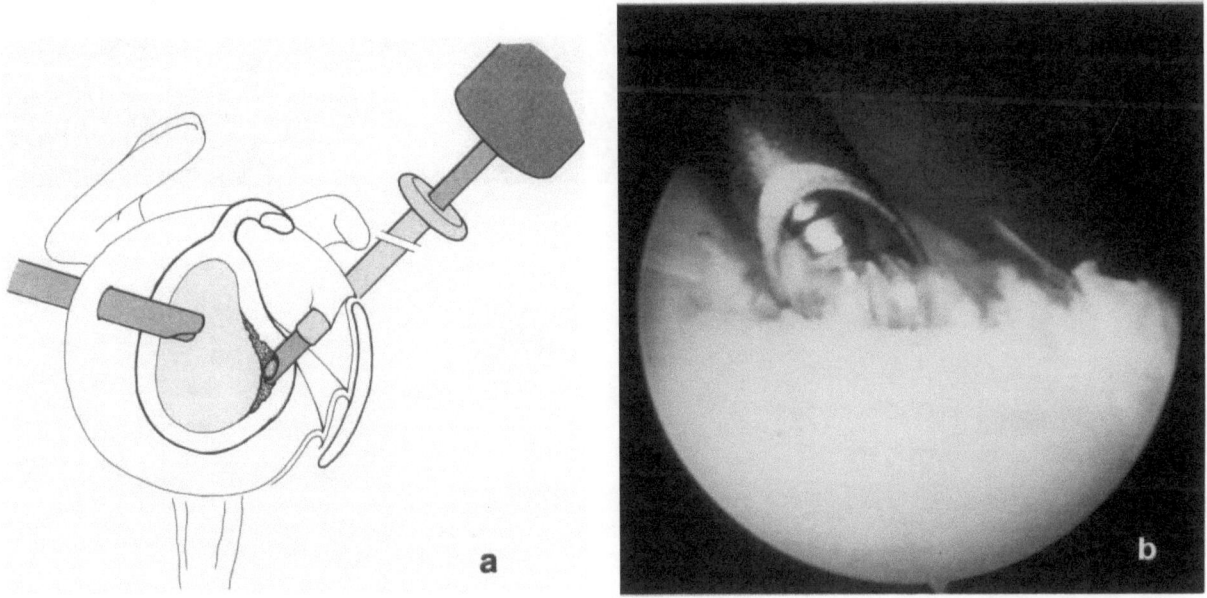

Fig. 95. Abrasion of glenoid rim. **a** Creating a groove with arthroplasty burr; **b** corresponding intraoperative picture

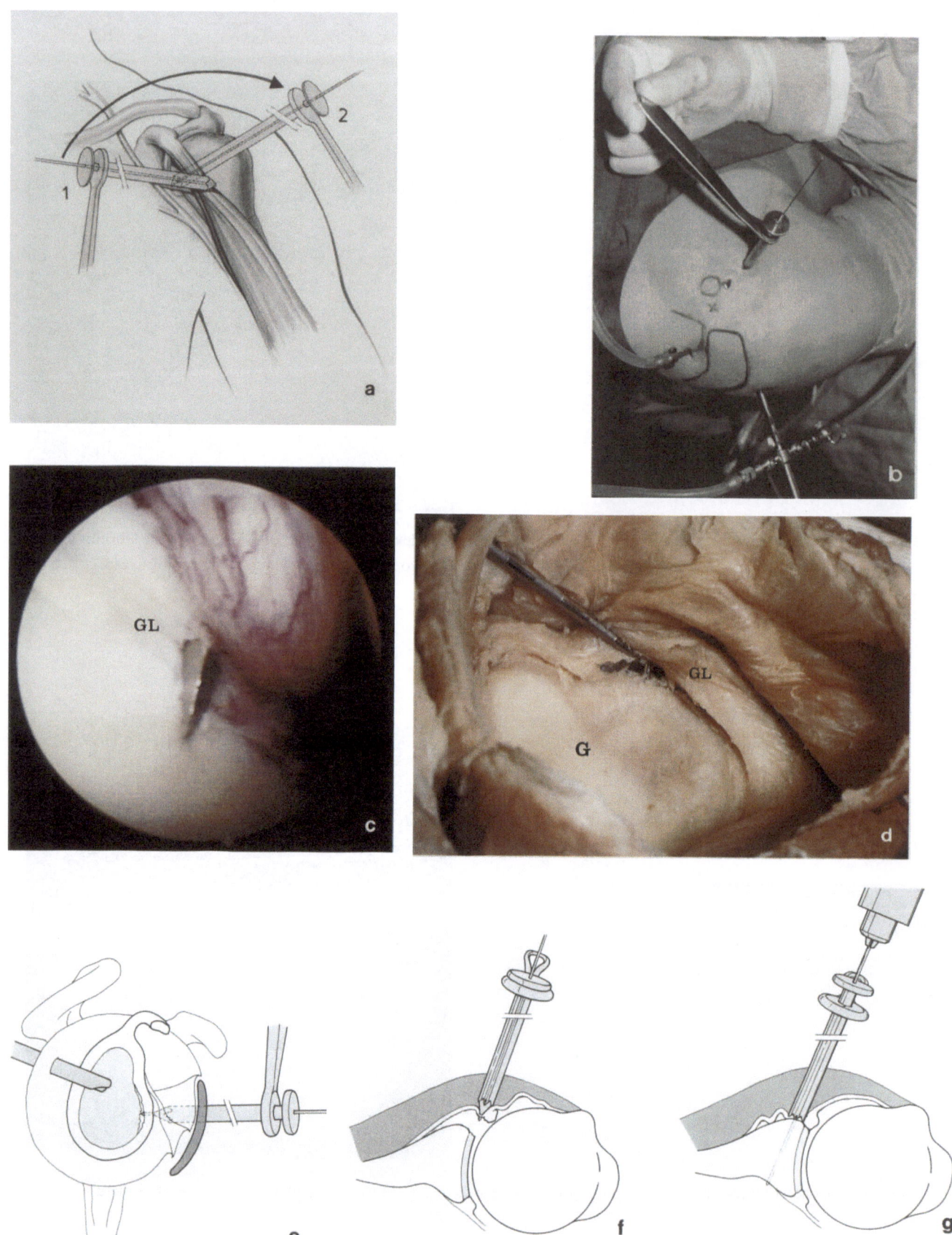

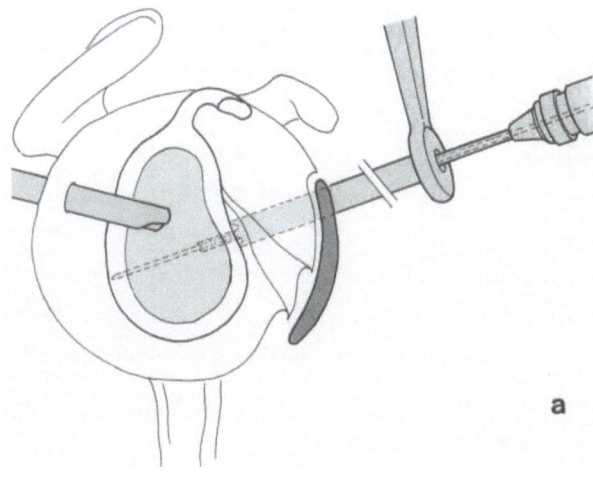

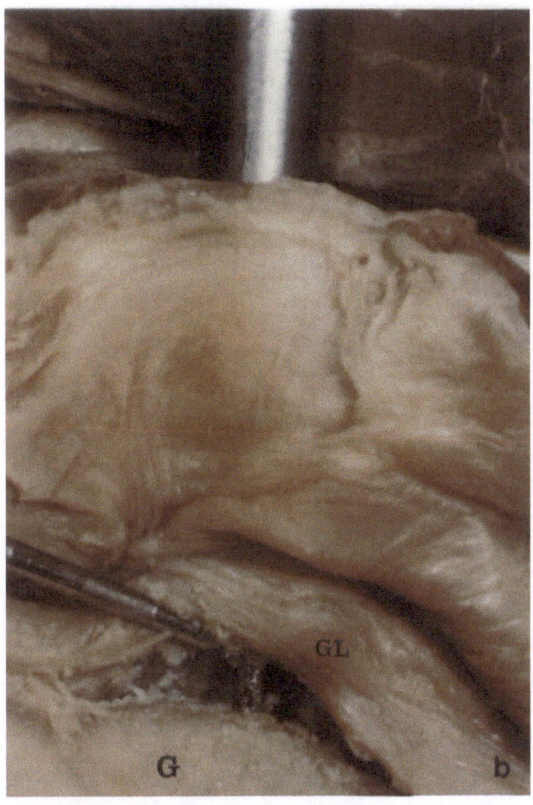

Fig. 97. Drilling with cannulated drill. **a** Schematic drawing. **b** Anatomical specimen. Glenoid labrum (*GL*) lifted from glenoid rim by means of the probe (inserted via antero-superior portal). *G* Glenoid

Fig. 96. Introduction of the trocar sheath, spearing and reduction of glenoid labrum. **a** Introduction of the cannula with the blunt trocar via the antero-inferior portal. First the cannula is directed dorsolaterally until it meets bony resistance (humeral head) (*1*), then the direction is changed dorsomedially toward the glenoid rim (*2*). **b** Trocar sheath with drill guide and guide wire introduced via antero-inferior portal. **c** Intraoperative picture with perforated glenoid labrum (*GL*). **d** Anatomical specimen; guide wire under vision; elevation of mobilized glenoid labrum (*GL*) with probe (inserted through antero-superior portal). *G* Glenoid. **e** Sagittal section; **f** transverse section. **g** Guide wire drilled into the opposite cortex. (Note: After drilling in the guide wire, it has to be cut slightly above the edge of the trocar sheath!)

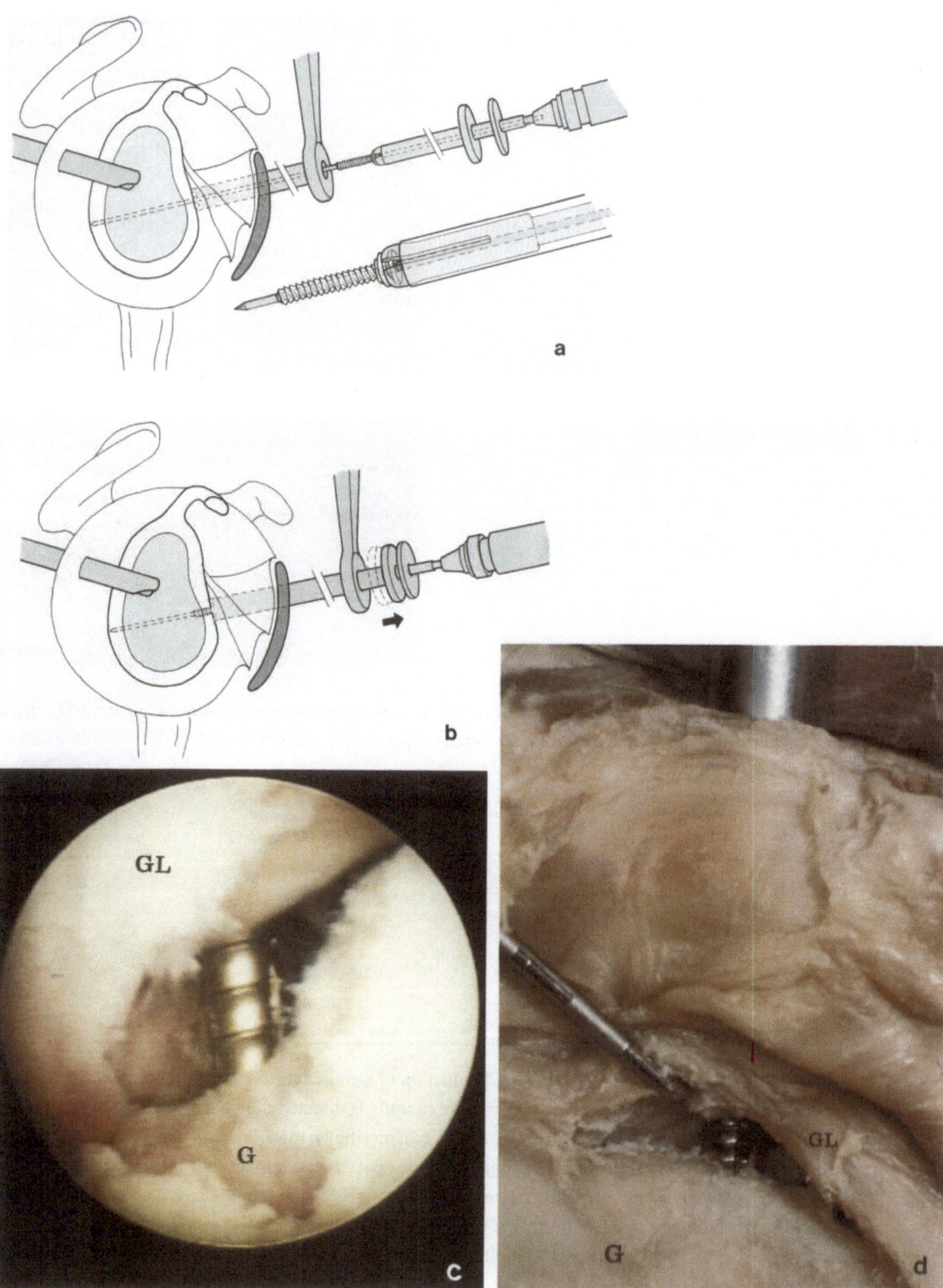

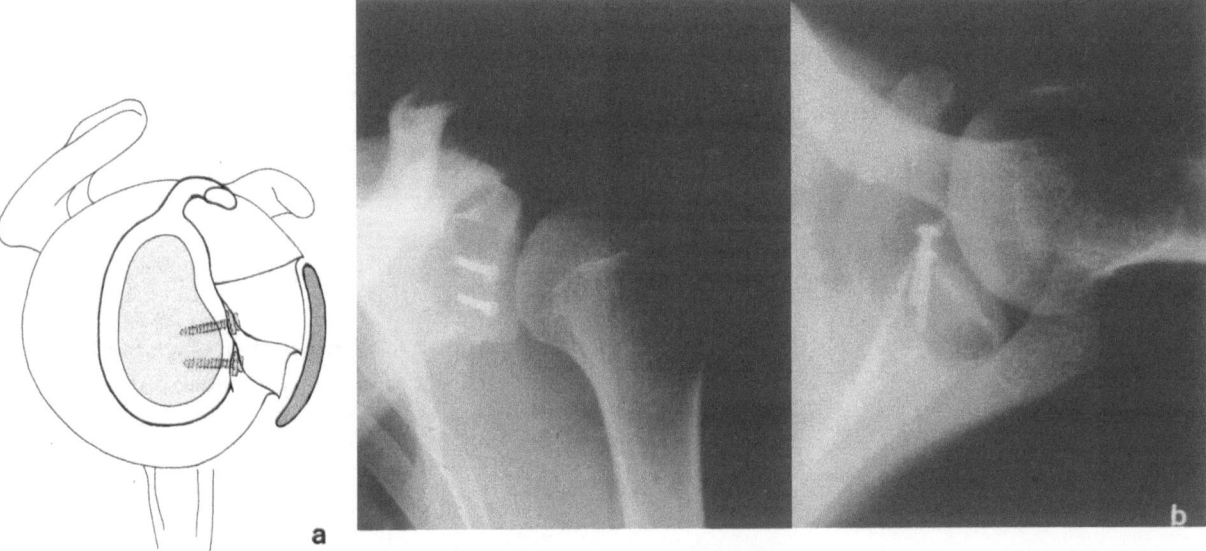

Fig. 99. Labrum fixed to glenoid rim extraarticularly by means of two screws. **a** Schematic drawing. **b** Postoperative roentgenogram

(3) Guide wire.   The 1 mm K-wire is very thin and may break if it is bent. Therefore, it should be carefully protected by the cannula. At the end of operation it should not be removed by means of the drill but by grasping it with a flat nose pliers at the posterior end and hammering it out or levering it out via the reinserted cannulated blunt trocar.

Arthroscopic extraarticular screw fixation of fractures of the glenoid rim

This technique is only feasible in cases of fresh fractures of the glenoid rim.

Technique

After thorough irrigation of the hemarthrosis, the probe is used for initial reduction of the fragment via the antero-superior portal. Through the antero-inferior portal (mind the musculocutaneous nerve!) the blunt trocar (drill guide) is advanced through the subscapularis muscle in the same manner as already described and the fragment is pressed onto the glenoid rim with the serrated end of the trocar sheath. Fine reduction of the fragment is performed by manipulation with the probe from the inside and the trocar sheath and/or drill guide from

◄──

Fig. 98. Introduction of screw over guide wire. **a** Screw locked in the tension plier. **b** After tightening the screw a few threads, retraction of tension sheath for loosening of the screw. **c** Intraoperative picture. View of screw through elevated glenoid labrum (*GL*), cartilage destroyed at glenoid rim. **d** Corresponding anatomical specimen. *GL* Glenoid labrum; *G* glenoid

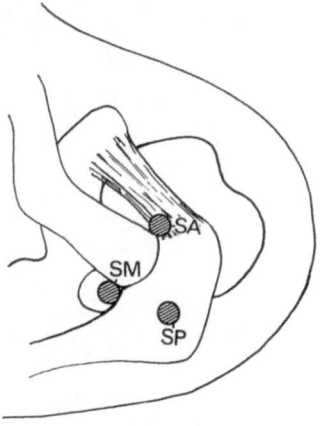

Fig. 100. Superior portals for arthroscopic screw fixation of a S.L.A.P. lesion; *SP* supero-posterior portal; *SA* supero-anterior portal; *SM* supero-medial portal

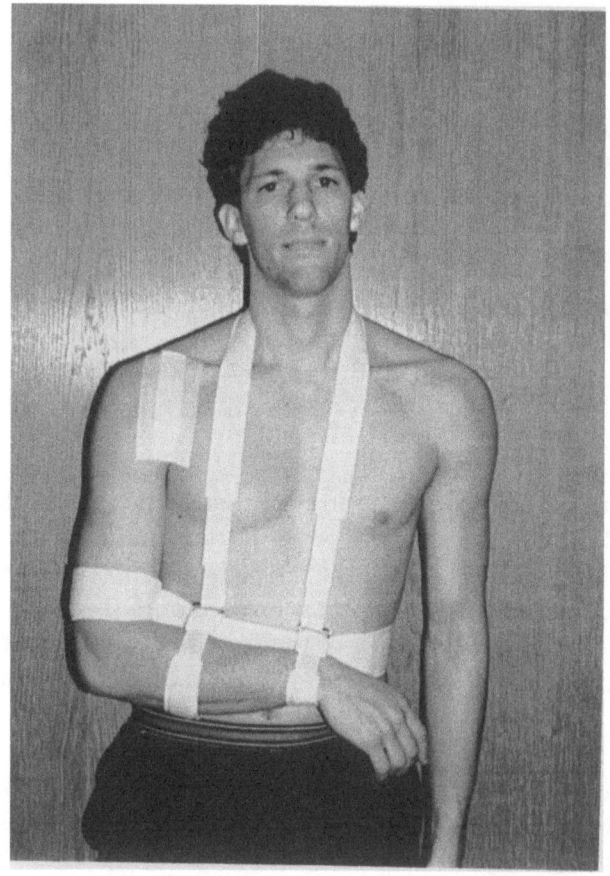

Fig. 101. Light shoulder bandage (according to Resch)

the outside. Screw fixation is performed in an extraarticular fashion. After adequate reduction has been achieved, the blunt trocar (drill guide) is advanced until it protrudes slightly into the joint. A 1 mm K-wire is advanced through the drill guide until it perforates the capsule immediately lateral to the fragment. This is done only to get better information about the position of the drill guide in relation to the fragment. Then the K-wire is withdrawn slightly and the drill guide shifted medially so that it is placed on the fragment. The 1 mm K-wire is drilled in through the fragment and the far cortex.

The remainder of the procedure is the same as already described above.

Arthroscopic screw fixation of a S.L.A.P. lesion

This lesion was first described by Snyder and collaborators in 1990 [30]. It is a lesion of the glenoid labrum which is located at the superior pole of the glenoid (superior labrum both anterior and posterior). In some of these cases the labrum together with the origin of the long head of the biceps tendon are detached, which is associated with an unstable anchor of the biceps (type II according to the classification of Snyder [30]). The refixation of this lesion is difficult to perform with the usual open methods as it is obstructed by the acromion. Even with arthroscopic suture repair, refixation is not possible as the wires when drilled through would exit in the axilla. The only possibility for refixation of a S.L.A.P. lesion to date is either arthroscopic screw fixation, with the screw having to be removed arthroscopically after 12 weeks, or refixation using absorbable tacks (see Chap. 6.4).

(The first patient presenting with this kind of lesion was operated on in October 1988, two years before it was published by Snyder.)

Technique

The arthroscope is introduced into the joint via the posterior portal. Abrasion of the lesion is performed via the standard anterior portal (anterior middle portal, which is placed immediately lateral to the tip of the coracoid process) with the rasp and the motorized burr (3.2 mm burr). In the case of a predominantly antero-superior lesion, the portal for the trocar (drill guide) is located directly at the anterior end of the acromion. If the lesion is mainly postero-superior, possible avenues of access are probed with a 1.6 mm K-wire to see whether the acromion can be circumvented anteriorly or medially, as the size of the acromion varies greatly. If the acromion cannot be circumvented, a hole with a diameter of 7 mm must be drilled through the acromion (transacromial approach). The blunt trocar (drill guide) is advanced to the lesion at the superior glenoid pole through the supraspinatus muscle and the capsule (Fig. 100). Firstly, the glenoid labrum is picked up immediately posterior to the origin of the long biceps tendon by the tip of the 1 mm K-wire and reduced to its original site. Then the guide wire is drilled in deeply. After the guide wire has been overdrilled by the cannulated drill, the labrum is fixed to the glenoid rim by means of a screw and washer. Sometimes a second screw is inserted into the glenoid rim via the antero-superior portal or the portal at the antero-medial end of the acromion. Removal of the screw is performed in the same manner under arthroscopic control three months later (intraarticularly placed metal should always be removed).

Intraarticular removal of screws.   This can be done arthroscopically when the screws are placed intraarticularly even after the guide wire has been removed. Again, the screw is loosened a few turns with the screw driver so that the screw holder can be advanced along the shaft of the screw driver over the screw head (Fig. 92 c and d). The screw can now be loosened easily and removed from the joint through the trocar sheath.

Postoperative treatment

Recurrent shoulder dislocation and screw fixation of glenoid fragments

Initial postoperative management includes immobilization in a light shoulder bandage (Gell, Innsbruck) for two weeks (Fig. 101). Subsequently, flexion of the shoulder of up to 90° and full internal rotation, is permitted. The motion permitted should be demonstrated to the patient on his healthy shoulder. From the sixth week on, motion is allowed in all planes. Sporting activities are permitted from the 14th postoperative week, provided that the shoulder muscles are equally developed on both sides.

S.L.A.P. lesion

Because of the adherent long biceps tendon, the shoulder should be immobilized for a total of 4 to 6 weeks (depending on the stability of the fixation). In this time passive motion should be performed two times a week. Subsequently, active motion is allowed in all planes. Exercises with weights are not allowed until the 12th postoperative week. Regular roentgeno-graphic examinations check the position of the screw which should be removed after approximately 12 weeks.

Patient information

As the arthroscopic screw technique has only recently been developed, the patient should be made aware of this fact and also the possibility that arthroscopic surgery may prove too difficult and be abandoned in favor of an open procedure. The patient should also be informed of possible complications arising from placement of screws and the possible necessity of later removal of such implants. The risk of neurological and other complication should also be explained before an "informed consent" can be obtained.

6.4 Arthroscopic Bankart refixation with absorbable staples

H. Resch, G. Sperner, and K. Golser

Having found intraarticularly inserted metal implants to be unsatisfactory for the refixation of the labrum-capsule complex to the glenoid rim [18, 21], the use of absorbable staples seemed to provide an obvious alternative. In this hospital we have for the past 24 months been using absorbable staples manufactured from poly-gluconate (Suretac, Acufex) which were developed in cooperation with Warren [1]. As the staples used are shaped more like tacks, it seems more appropriate to refer to them as tacks. According to the manufacturer, these tacks maintain their shape up to 6 weeks after their insertion into the body but are completely absorbed after 6 months. This provides adequate time for the capsule and/or glenoid labrum to heal back onto the glenoid rim. The principle of the introduction of the tacks is similar to the screw fixation technique described in Chap. 6.3. As we are dealing with unthreaded tacks, they are not screwed into the drill-hole but driven in.

Indications

So far, the tacks have been inserted mostly using an intraarticular approach. The prerequisites for the use of these implants are therefore similar to those for the suturing technique (Chaps. 6.1 and 6.2). The labrum must be largely preserved in shape and continuity so that it can be used for the refixation of the capsule. As for all arthroscopic techniques, the bony glenoid rim should be intact. Also, patients with hyperlax joints should be managed with open surgery rather than arthroscopic methods. Indications for this technique are the following:

- Recurrent anterior dislocation and subluxation.
- Detachment of the labrum from the antero-superior glenoid rim in the course of an impingement syndrome [5, 23] (see also Chaps. 6.1 and 7.1).
- Labral detachments at the superior glenoid pole (S.L.A.P. lesion [30]; see also Chap. 6.3).

More recently absorbable tacks (instead of screws) were applied also for extraarticular refixation of the capsule according to the technique described in Chap. 6.3 But the number of cases is too small and the follow-up time too short for a definite evaluation.

Instrumentation

The cannulated implant is shaped like a tack and is 18 mm long. The head has a diameter of 6.5 mm and the shaft is 3.2 mm in diameter (Fig. 102). A trocar sheath with a blunt trocar is used to insert the implant as well as a 1 mm guide wire, a cannulated 3.2 mm drill (TriPointDrill), a cannulated handpiece, a drill adapter for machine drive and a cannulated driver (Suretac driver) (Fig. 103).

Recurrent dislocations and subluxations

Anesthesia and positioning are the same as for the previously described operative methods. This technique is usually performed under regional anesthesia (interscalene block; see Chap. 2) since a reduction of the arterial blood pressure is not required. In a few cases, regional anesthesia is combined with general anesthesia. The lateral as well as the half-sitting position can be used; we have come to favor the so-called beach-chair position [1, 29] (see Chap. 3). As in all other arthroscopic interventions, the arm is abducted to 30° and placed in a right-angled arthroscopic elbow brace to which a traction weight of 2 kg is attached.

Intraarticular technique

Beside the posterior portal which is located 1.5 cm medial and 1 cm inferior to the acromial angle, only the standard anterior portal is necessary. This is located directly lateral to the tip of the coracoid process. After the skin incision, the 7 mm trocar sheath is inserted together with the blunt trocar into the joint at the superior margin of the tendon of the subscapularis muscle (Fig. 104). A 7 mm plastic cannula may also be used as a sheath (Disposable Cannula, Acufex). Next, the glenoid labrum with the adherent capsule is mobilized with the shoulder elevator (Acufex) so that it can be reduced onto the glenoid rim while simultaneously tensing it in a cranial direction. The bony glenoid rim is roughened with the Bankart rasp (Acufex) and subsequently a 4.5 mm arthroplasty burr (Concept) is used to create a longitudinal groove (see also Chap. 6.3). Then the 1 mm guide wire is inserted into the cannulated drill until it protrudes a few millimeters beyond the end of the drill. They are inserted into the joint together and the previously mobilized labrum is speared with the tip of the guide wire, reduced onto the glenoid rim and tensed in a superior direction. After meeting a bony resistance, the wire is drilled in to the far cortex. The thin wire is supported by the drill during this procedure. When drilling in the wire, it must at least be 2 mm away from the glenoid articular surface, since the cartilage may otherwise become distorted when driving in the tacks. With the elbow bent at a right angle, the arm is externally rotated 30° to determine the correct position of the capsule. If the capsule is not tensed by this rotation, the inferior glenohumeral ligament should be partially incorporated in the repair. Next, a hole for the tack is drilled while observing the mark on the shaft to avoid drilling out the wire (Fig. 105). When using a drill which is not entirely cannulated, the wire has to be shortened before drilling. If using a completely cannulated drill (Zimmer) a special drilling accessory can be used, which permits the guide wire and the drill to be locked in place alternately. Thus the guide wire can be placed and the drill-hole made in one step. After removing the drill, a tack is advanced over the guide wire and driven in with the Suretac driver under arthroscopic control (Fig. 106a and b). After inspecting the refixation of the labrum with the probe, the guide wire is removed. Usually, a second tack is inserted 1 cm from the first, and sometimes also a third tack (Fig. 107). If multiple tacks are to be used, their locations must be planned at the start of the procedure.

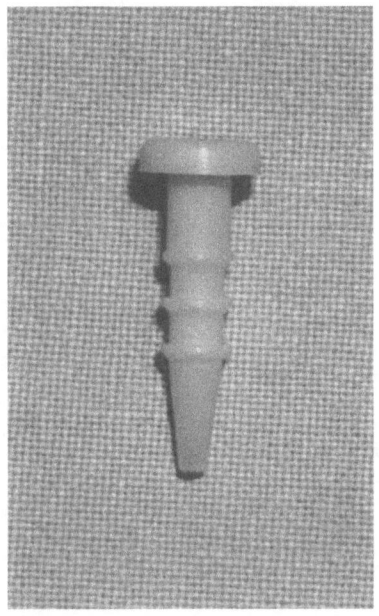 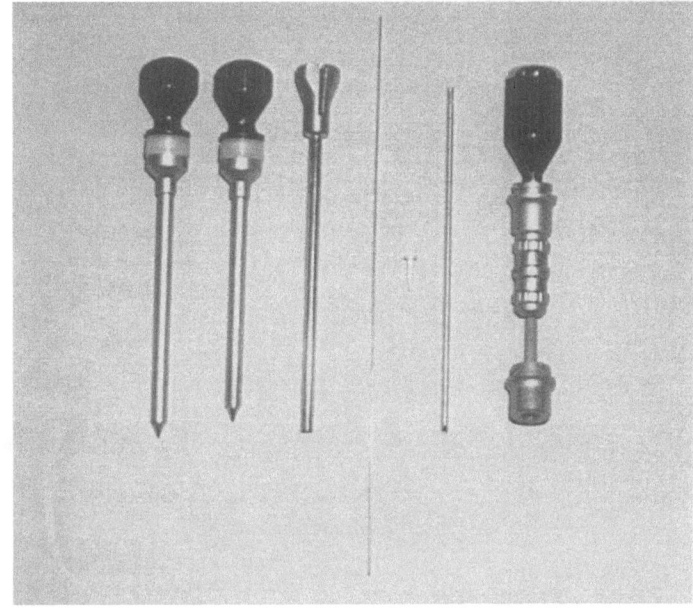

Fig. 102   Fig. 103

Fig. 102. Suretac

Fig. 103. Instrumentation; from left to right: trocar cannulas of different lengths with inserted trocar, Suretac driver, 1 mm guide wire, Suretac, drill, handle with locking mechanism (Universal Chuck), adaptor for drill

Extraarticular technique

The indications for this technique are the same as described for the extraarticular screw fixation technique (Chap. 6.3). As in the screw fixation technique the same anterior portals (antero-superior and antero-inferior portal) are used. But our experience is not sufficient to date to render definite results.

Hazards and complications

The guide wire must be drilled in at a safe distance (at least 2 mm) from the glenoid articular surface. When drilling the hole for the tack, the articular cartilage should be watched closely in order to prevent the thicker drill from damaging the cartilage.

The guide wire should not be removed by means of the drill but by grasping it with a flat nose pliers at the posterior end and hammering it out. The thin wire might have been bent during the different steps of the procedure and therefore be prone to break if removing it using the machine.

With the exception of two broken guide wires during removal, no peri- or postoperative complications have been recorded at the time of writing.

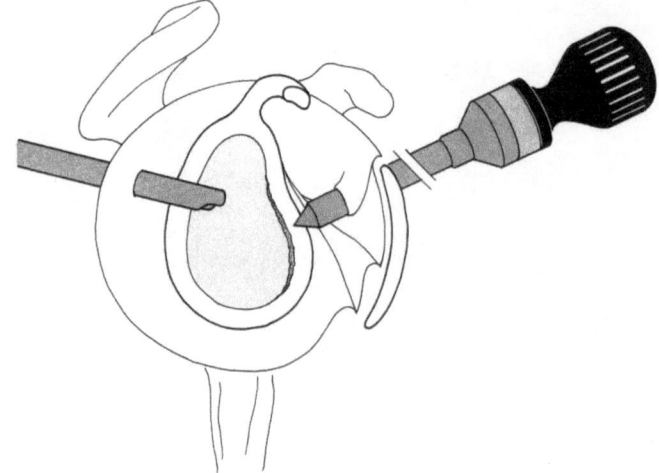

Fig. 104. Insertion of trocar cannula via anterior standard portal

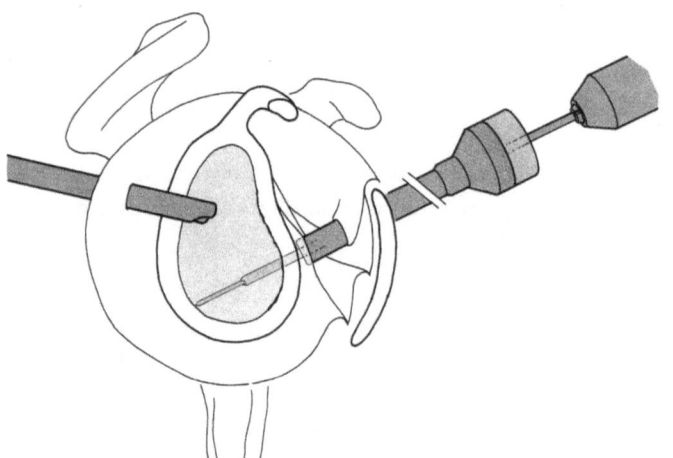

Fig. 105. After picking up the labrum, drilling in the guide wire to the opposite cortex and subsequent drilling with cannulated drill

Refixation of the glenoid labrum at the superior glenoid pole (S.L.A.P. lesion, Type II)

This lesion presents a pathological change of the glenoid labrum at the superior pole of the glenoid, where the tendon of the long head of the biceps originates (S.L.A.P.). For the first time it was described by Snyder et al. in 1990 [30]. He classified the lesion into four types. Type II is of special interest to us, because in this type the labrum together with the anchor of the long head of the biceps tendon is completely detached from the bony rim of the upper pole of the glenoid (Fig. 108). This means that the origin of the long biceps tendon is destabilized. We think that type II should be refixed. We performed the first refixation of a S.L.A.P. lesion in October 1988 by open surgery, since we have developed an arthroscopic technique we did it by arthroscopy.

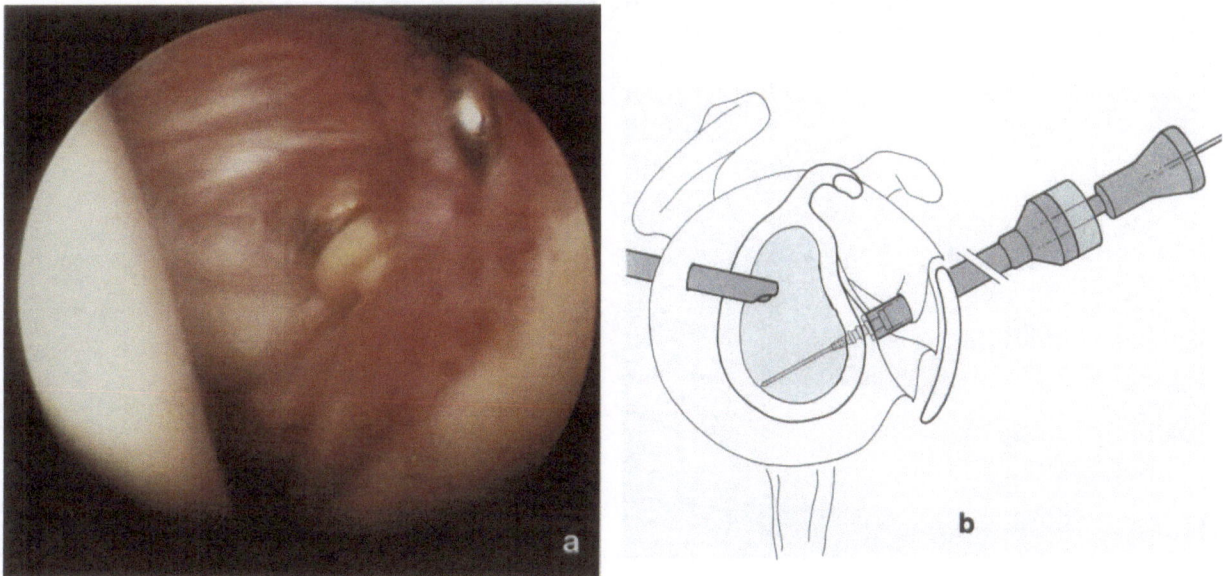

Fig. 106. a Refixation of a detached and inflamed labrum; Suretac is almost driven in by the Suretac-driver.
b Drawing: Suretac driver used to insert and drive in Suretac

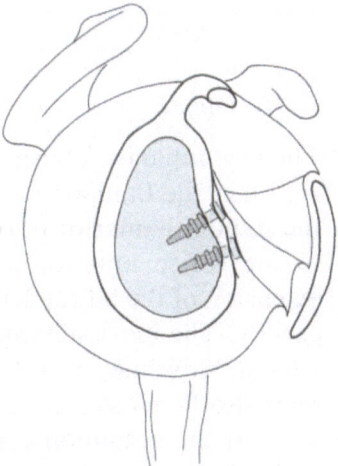

Fig. 107. Labrum-capsule complex fixed with two Suretacs

This type of labral detachment produces impingement-like symptoms. The palm-up test is positive and the apprehension test [13, 14] is most often painful but not positive. Often the patients are throwing athletes who consult the physician because they experience pain when throwing. There are usually no signs of subluxation. Open as well as arthroscopic refixation of the detachment is difficult due to the obstruction of the acromion process (see also Chap. 6.3).

In the first 5 cases the labrum was refixed by screws (see Chap. 6.3) and in the last 10 cases by absorbable tacks.

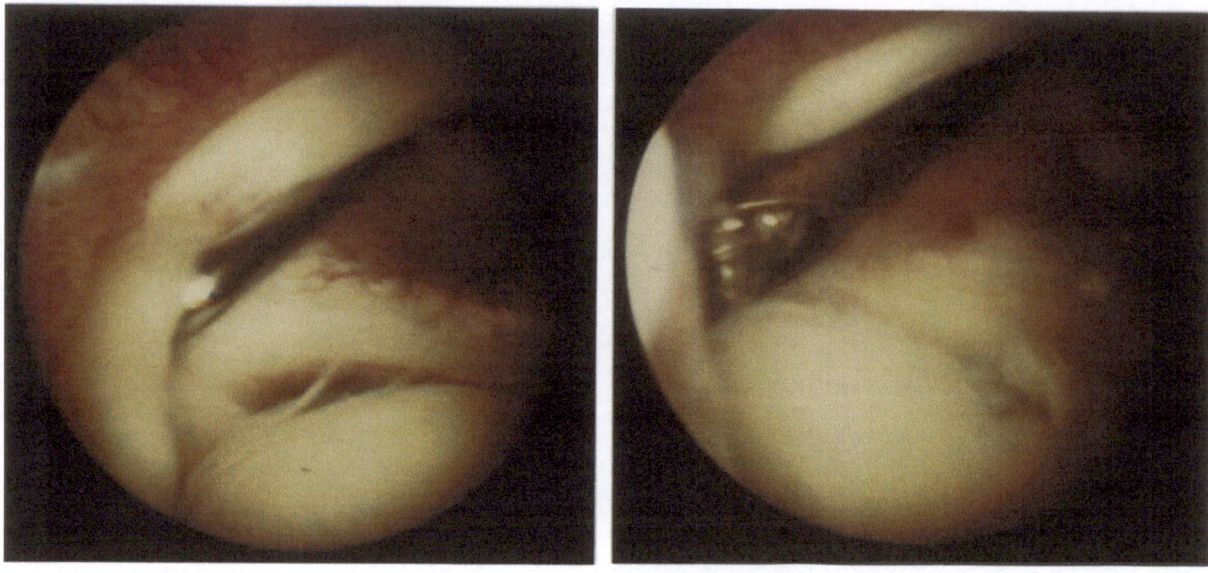

Fig. 108   Fig. 109

Fig. 108. S.L.A.P. lesion type II. Detached labrum together with the long biceps tendon lifted up by the probe

Fig. 109. Abrasion of the bony rim with the burr

Technique

The technique is very similar to the technique already described in Chap. 6.3.

First, the Bankart rasp (Acufex) and then the 3.2 mm arthroplasty burr are inserted via the standard anterior portal and used to abrade the glenoid rim thoroughly (Fig. 109). Due to the varied anterior and lateral extension of the acromion, and the varied posterior extension of the labral detachment, the portal to the superior glenoid pole cannot be defined exactly. The most suitable access to the superior glenoid pole should be determined with a 1.6 mm Kirschner wire. It can often be found directly at the end of the acromion. The portal may also be most convenient at the medial border of the acromion slightly behind the AC joint. If the acromion cannot be circumvented, a hole with a diameter of 7 mm is drilled through the acromion (Chap. 6.3, Fig. 100). The drill-hole should be placed at the midpoint of the acromion in order to avoid fractures. This portal should only be used as a last resort. The trocar sheath with the blunt trocar is inserted through the supraspinatus muscle and the capsule. The 1 mm guide wire is inserted into the joint together with the drill, which serves as a support for the wire, and subsequently the glenoid labrum is picked up slightly behind the origin of the long biceps tendon and reduced onto the superior glenoid pole (Fig. 110a–d). The wire is drilled deeply into the bony glenoid. The probe is inserted via the standard anterior portal and used to elevate the labrum slightly so as to facilitate the placement of the guide wire. During the drilling procedure, beware of distortion of the cartilage. The remainder of the procedure, driving in the tacks, does not differ from the one

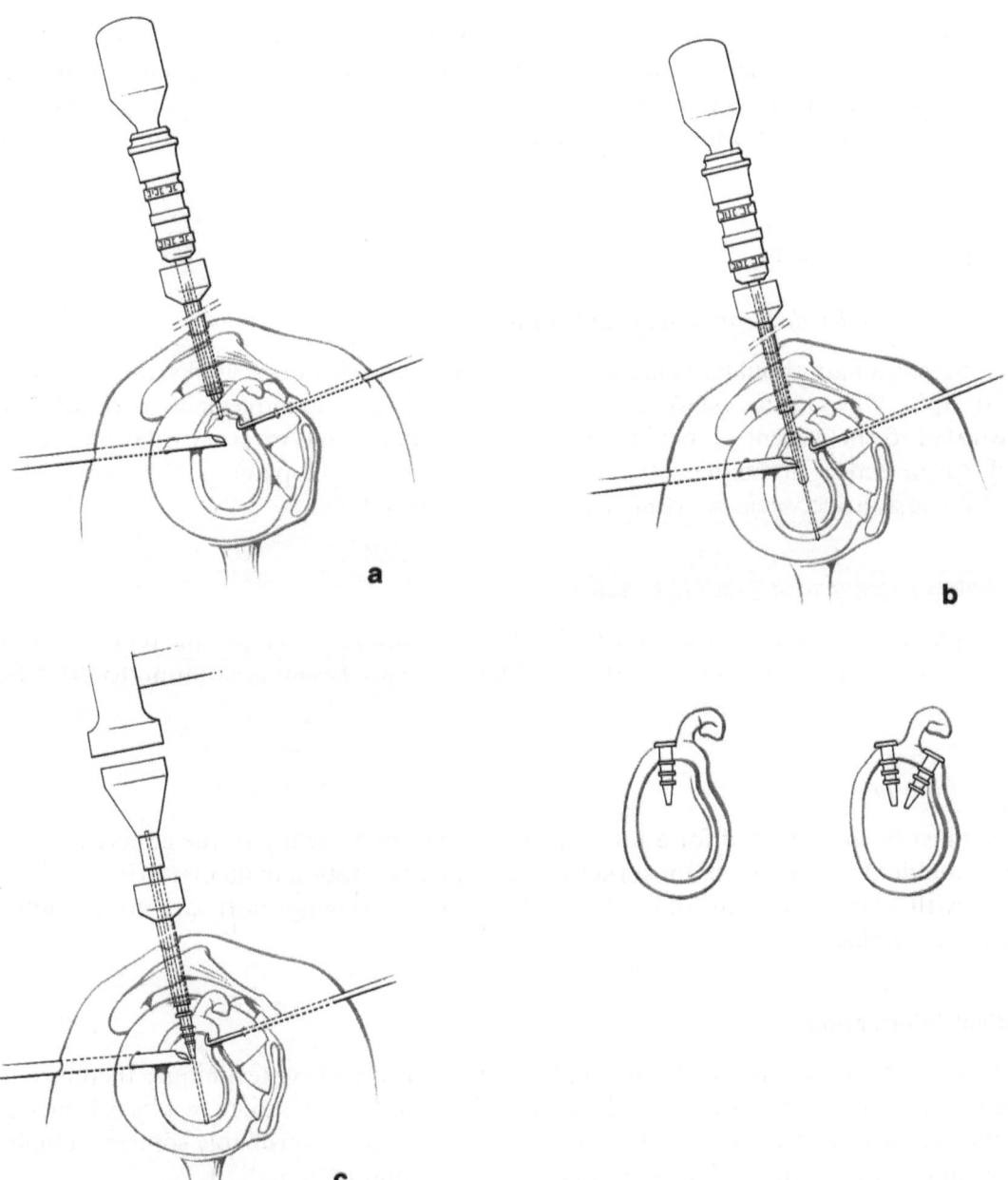

Fig. 110. Technique of arthroscopic refixation of a S.L.A.P. lesion type II. **a** Introduction of the cannula with the blunt trocar using the transacromial approach; the glenoid labrum is picked up by the tip of the guide wire immediately posterior to the origin of the long biceps tendon; the guide wire is guided by the cannulated burr or by the cannulated blunt trocar; the wire is drilled in deeply. **b** Overdrilling of the guide wire with the cannulated drill. **c** Insertion of the biodegradable tack (Suretac) with Suretac driver and hammer. **d** The detached labrum is refixed either by one tack, which is always placed immediately posterior to the long head of the biceps (left), or in cases with a larger lesion by two tacks. The second tack is always inserted anteriorly to the biceps tendon using an anterior or antero-superior approach

described above. Depending on the extent of the lesion, a second tack may be inserted from an antero-superior approach (standard anterior portal or antero-superior portal; see Chaps. 6.1–3) (Fig. 110d). As there is very little space available at the superior glenoid pole, the placement of the tacks must be determined exactly prior to the procedure being performed.

Postoperative treatment

Recurrent shoulder dislocation and subluxation

Postoperatively, a light shoulder bandage is applied and worn for three weeks. Subsequently, flexion of up to 90° and free internal rotation are permitted (the movements permitted are demonstrated to the patient on his healthy arm). Abduction and external rotation are not allowed. At the end of the sixth postoperative week, motion in all planes is permitted. After the 14th postoperative week, sporting activities are allowed.

Antero-superior detachment of the labrum

The postoperative treatment is the same as for shoulder dislocation. After the removal of the shoulder bandage, impingement exercises (see Chap. 7.1) are begun in addition to the other exercises.

S.L.A.P. lesion

The arm must be immobilized for a total of four to six weeks owing to the adherent biceps tendon (shoulder bandage; Gell, Innsbruck). Subsequently, motion in all planes is permitted. Exercises with weights are only allowed after 12 weeks. Throwing sports are not permitted until after 24 weeks.

Patient information

The refixation of the labrum with absorbable tacks is a very new technique, therefore no long-term follow-up results are available to date. Even though the early results are encouraging, the patient must be informed that the risk of a recurrence is probably somewhat higher than for an open procedure. This may necessitate a second intervention.

6.5 Evaluation of the individual arthroscopic Bankart refixation techniques and our own method

H. Resch

In the university hospital of Innsbruck, arthroscopic refixation of the labrum-capsule complex (in various areas of the glenoid), was performed in 178 patients. Suture repair was performed in 51 cases, screw fixation was applied in 85 cases, and the technique using absorbable tacks (Suretac, Acufex) in 42 cases. The refixation procedure with absorbable tacks was carried out in the course of an FDA study.

Arthroscopic Bankart suture repair

This technique was used on 51 patients. Sixteen patients underwent arthroscopic refixation of the labrum after initial dislocation, 14 because of recurrent anterior subluxation and 9 patients due to recurrent dislocation. Twelve patients with an impingement syndrome had a detachment of the glenoid labrum from the antero-superior aspect of the glenoid (secondary impingement). After a mean follow-up period of 24 months (6 to 48 months) all patients who had undergone surgery following initial dislocation were stable. Of the patients with recurrent subluxations, one patient continued to show unchanged symptoms as well as a positive apprehension test. Among the 9 patients with recurrent dislocation there was no postoperative recurrence. One patient, however, demonstrated symptoms of subluxation. Thus the patients with recurrent dislocation or subluxation have a remaining postoperative instability rate of 8.6%. In 72% of all patients with instability, the postoperative range of motion was equal on both sides, in 20% external rotation was reduced by less than 10° and in 8% by more than 10°.

Of the 12 patients with antero-superior lesions, refixation effected a considerable improvement or disappearance of the impingement complaints in 8 cases (66%). In retrospective analysis, the glenoid labrum in the remaining 4 patients was probably too damaged at the time of operation to allow for successful refixation. Three of these 4 patients later underwent subacromial decompression with successful results.

Advantages and disadvantages of the technique

A quick and relatively simple technique.

The glenoid labrum should be largely preserved in shape and continuity so that it can be used for refixation of the capsule.

Due to the sutures exiting posteriorly under the skin, immobilization is required for a period of 3 to 4 weeks.

If the Bankart needles are drilled out too far superiorly and medially, the suprascapularis nerve may be damaged.

In case of a marked periarticular edema, the sutures may become loose after the swelling has receded (knots have to be tied as deep down as possible).

Arthroscopic three-point Bankart suture repair

In the series described by Habermeyer, refixation of the labrum-capsule complex was performed on 82 patients because of unidirectional anterior instability. 22 patients had recurrent shoulder dislocation and 60 patients recurrent subluxation. After a mean follow-up period of 16 months (4 to 36 months), 3 patients with recurrent shoulder dislocation had a postoperative recurrence. Of the 60 patients with recurrent subluxation, 7 patients continued to have subluxation symptoms on follow-up examination as well as a positive apprehension test. The postoperative instability rate is thus 12%. The mobility at the time of the follow-up examination was equal on both shoulders in 80% of the cases, in 12% of the cases external rotation was limited by less than 10° and in 8% of the cases by more than 10°.

Advantages and disadvantages of the technique compared with the Bankart suturing technique mentioned above

The sutures are not tied posteriorly under the skin, which shortens the period of immobilization. Furthermore, the sutures do not become loose after the periarticular edema of the soft tissue has disappeared.

As mentioned in the technique described above, the glenoid labrum should be preserved in shape and continuity so as to enable adequate refixation of the capsule.

As the sutures are tied anteriorly by means of a knot pusher, this technique is more time-consuming and more demanding technically.

Damage to the suprascapularis nerve is possible as the pins are drilled through posteriorly.

Arthroscopic Bankart screw fixation technique

This technique was applied in 85 patients. In the first 32 patients, screw fixation of the glenoid labrum was performed by an intraarticular technique. Due to a screw loosening rate of 13%, only the extraarticular technique was used in the following 52 patients. In one patient with a SLAP lesion, intraarticular refixation with a screw was performed at a later date. In 52 patients with extraarticular screw fixation there was no evidence of screw loosening.

Of the 85 patients 59 had a unidirectional anterior instability: in 51 cases there was recurrent dislocation and in 8 cases recurrent subluxation. In the remaining patients, 8 had fresh fractures of the antero-inferior glenoid rim, 13 had a detachment of the glenoid labrum on the antero-superior aspect of the glenoid combined with the symptoms of an impingement syndrome (secondary impingement) and in 5 patients a S.L.A.P. lesion was present.

Extraarticular screw fixation was performed in 52 of the 59 patients with anterior instability. Of the patients with extraarticular screw fixation technique (average 15 months, range 3 to 30 months) the recurrency rate was 3.8% (2 cases). In all patients with recurrent subluxations the subluxation symptoms had disappeared and the apprehension test was negative. Twenty-seven of the 52 patients with extraarticular refixation technique achieved equal mobility on both sides, in 16 patients external rotation was limited by less than 10° and in 9 patients by more than 10°.

Of the 8 patients with screw fixation of an antero-inferior glenoid rim fragment (in 3 cases intraarticular and in 5 cases extraarticular fixation), 7 patients achieved stable and equally mobile shoulders. In the 8th patient external rotation was limited by 15° as compared to the contralateral shoulder.

Of the 13 patients with screw fixation of an antero-superior detachment of the labrum (in all cases intraarticular screw fixation), 8 patients (62%) showed a marked improvement of the impingement symptoms. Of the remaining 5 patients, 3 underwent arthroscopic subacromial decompression at a later date.

Of the 5 patients with screw fixation of a S.L.A.P. lesion (in 1 case via a transacromial approach), 4 have since had their screws removed arthroscopically. Two of the 4 patients returned to their overhead sports activities after 5 and 8 months, respectively. One patient has experienced no pain relief and the other patient only slight improvement. At the time of writing, it was too early to evaluate the remaining patient.

Our experience leads us to advocate the extraarticular screw fixation method, avoiding the placement of metal within the joint. If intraarticular screw fixation cannot be avoided, regular roentgenographic examinations should be undertaken and an early arthroscopic removal of the screw considered.

Advantages and disadvantages of the extraarticular Bankart screw fixation compared with the suturing techniques

This technique allows the refixation of the labrum-capsule complex in the center of the Bankart lesion. It permits the shortening of an enlarged capsule, as well.

The success of the technique does not depend on the state of the glenoid labrum as screw fixation of the capsule itself to the glenoid rim is performed extraarticularly.

It can also be used in cases of fresh glenoid fractures.

It is technically demanding (two experienced arthroscopists required).

Relatively short immobilization for a period of up to 2 weeks; only a S.L.A.P. lesion requires an immobilization period of 4 to 6 weeks.

Screw fixation of detachments of the labrum to the antero-superior aspect of the glenoid can generally not be performed extraarticularly because of the subscapularis bursa. In these cases, the suturing technique or the technique using absorbable tacks is preferred.

The insertion of metal into the body may lead to a variety of complications.

The thin guide wire (1 mm) may be bent and can break if it is not carefully protected by the cannula.

Bankart refixation with absorbable staples (Suretac, Acufex)

To date, a total of 42 patients have had this type of refixation performed in the course of an FDA study. There were 27 patients with recurrent anterior shoulder dislocation and/or subluxation, 5 patients with antero-superior detachment of the glenoid labrum and 10 patients with a S.L.A.P. lesion. With the exception of 8 patients in all other cases the tacks were implanted by an intraarticular technique.

Recurrent anterior shoulder dislocation and/or subluxation

- Intraarticular technique. Of the 19 patients in this group, 17 had recurrent dislocation whilst 2 had recurrent subluxation. With a mean follow-up of 13 months (3 to 24 months), there has been one recurrence to date. One patient who underwent surgery because of a recurrent shoulder dislocation has had a positive apprehension test 6 months after the operation and complains of the feeling of instability. All the other patients have a negative apprehension test. With the exception of 4 patients, all have regained full range of motion.
- Extraarticular technique. Eight patients with recurrent dislocation have been operated on to date (average 6 months, range, 1 to 12 months). After this short time no redislocation has occurred.

Antero-superior detachment of the labrum

The 5 patients showed a definite impingement syndrome on physical examination and a strongly positive subacromial LA test. In all 5 patients the glenoid labrum was completely detached antero-superiorly but preserved in shape and continuity. Furthermore, 4 patients had an associated local synovitis in the antero-superior aspect of the capsule (see also Chap. 6.3). The glenoid labrum was reattached but in all cases no additional acromioplasty was performed. Postoperatively, all patients participated in a muscle strengthening program (see Chap. 7.1). At present, after a mean period of 13 months (3 to 24 months), 4 patients showed a distinct improvement of their symptoms. One patient has failed to show any marked improvement. In this case acromioplasty was performed 5 months postoperatively.

S.L.A.P. lesion

In all 10 patients the glenoid labrum was completely detached from antero-superior to postero-superior and, due to the long biceps tendon, protruded superiorly like a bucket-handle. In 2 of the 10 patients, refixation was performed via a transacromial approach. In 4 of the 10 patients 2 tacks were introduced (one from a superior approach and one from antero-superiorly); in the remaining patients one tack was sufficient for the refixation. At present, after a mean period of 12 months (5 to 23 months) all symptoms have disappeared in 5 patients. One of the patients, a handball player (throwing arm), has improved but has not regained his previous level of performance. Two other patients have experienced no improvement. In the remaining two patients time is to short for evaluation.

Advantages and disadvantages of the Bankart refixation with absorbable staples compared with the previously described refixation techniques

Relatively simple technique. The absorbability of the staples has distinct advantages over the metal implants. No sutures have to be tied posteriorly over the muscles and/or no time-consuming and demanding tying with knot pusher from an anterior approach.

A disadvantage compared with the screw fixation technique is the fact that the labrum must be largely preserved in shape and continuity to successfully perform the intraarticular techniques.

Our own method in the case of recurrent shoulder dislocation and subluxation

The prerequisite for an arthroscopic stabilization of the unidirectional shoulder dislocation is a glenoid which is largely preserved in shape, size and inclination. Dislocation patients with old glenoid rim fractures require open surgery. Also, patients with marked joint hypermobility are not candidates for arthroscopic surgery because the capsular redundancy should be corrected in an open procedure.

Based on our experience with various intra- and extraarticular refixation techniques we prefer to treat patients with a Bankart lesion (recurrent dislocation and subluxation) by an extraarticular refixation technique (screws, sometimes sutures, and more recently also absorbable tacks). Only in the rare cases with a detached but preserved labrum and not enlarged capsule (e.g., subluxation) an intraarticular technique (sutures, absorbable tacks) is applied.

In patients with a detachment of the labrum at the antero-superior or superior aspect of the glenoid an intraarticular technique using suture or absorbable tacks is preferred.

In other words, an extraarticular refixation technique is preferred in the lower half of the glenoid, whereas an intraarticular technique is given preference in the upper half.

References

1. Altcheck DW, Warren RF, Skyhar MJ (1990) Shoulder arthroscopy. In: Rockwood JR, Matsen FA (eds) The shoulder. WB Saunders, Philadelphia, pp 258–277
2. Altcheck DW, Skyhar MJ, Warren RF (1989) Shoulder arthroscopy for shoulder instability. In: Barr JS (ed) Instructional course lectures. Am Acad Orthop Surg 28:187–198
3. Andrews JR, Angelo RI (1988) Arthroscopy for the throwing athlete. Techniques Orthop 3:75–81
4. Andrews JR, Broussard TS, Carson WG (1989) Arthroscopy of the shoulder in the management of partial tears of the rotator cuff: a preliminary report. Arthroscopy 1:117–121
5. Andrews JR, Carson WG, McLeod WD (1985) Glenoid labrum tears related to the long head of the biceps. Am J Sports Med 13:337–341
6. Andrews JR, Carson WG, Ortega K (1984) Arthroscopy of the shoulder. Am J Sports Med 12:1–7
7. Bankart ASB (1928) The pathology and treatment of recurrent dislocation of the shoulder joint. Br J Surg 26:23–29
8. Bankart ASB (1923) Recurrent or habitual dislocation of the shoulder joint. Br Med J 2:1123–1133
9. Berner W, Tscherne H (1986) Die Arthroskopie des Schultergelenkes. Orthop Praxis 22:85
10. Bunnell ST, Böhler J (1958) Chirurgie der Hand, 1. German edn. Maudrich, Wien

11. Caspari RB (1988) Arthroscopic reconstruction for anterior shoulder instability. Techniques Orthop 3:59–66

12. Gächter A, Kählin L (1987) Diagnostische Arthroskopie des Schultergelenkes. In: Gächter A (eds) Arthroskopie der Schulter. Enke, Stuttgart, pp 31–37 [Hofer A, Glinz W (eds) Fortschritte in der Arthroskopie, vol 3]

13. Gerber C (1984) Differentialdiagnostische Aspekte posttraumatischer Schulterschmerzen. Unfallheilkunde 87:357–362

14. Gerber C, Ganz R (1984) Clinical assessment of instability of the shoulder. J Bone Joint Surg [Br] 66:551–556

15. Glötzer W, Benedetto PP, Künzel KH, Gaber O (1987) Technik der arthroskopischen Limbusrefixation. In: Gächter A (ed) Arthroskopie der Schulter. Enke, Stuttgart, pp 63–66 [Hofer H, Glinz W (eds) Fortschritte in der Arthroskopie, vol 3]

16. Habermeyer P, Schuller U (1990) Die Bedeutung des Labrum glenoidale für die Stabilität des Schultergelenkes. Unfallchirurg 93:19–26

17. Haniel H (1990) Physikalische Therapie im Rahmen der postoperativen Behandlung. In: Habermeyer P, Krueger P, Schweiberer L (eds) Schulterchirurgie. Urban & Schwarzenberg, München, pp 263–276

18. Hawkins RB (1989) Arthroscopic stapling repair for shoulder instability: a retrospective study of 50 cases. Arthroscopy 5:122–128

19. Johnson LL (1986) Shoulder arthroscopy. In: Klein EA, Falk KH, O'Brien T (eds) Arthroscopic surgery, principles and practice. CV Mosby, St Louis, pp 1301–1445

20. Johnson LL (1987) The shoulder joint. An arthroscopist's perspective of anatomy and pathology. Clin Orthop 223:113–125

21. Matthews LS, Vetter WL, Oweida SJ, Spearman J, Helfet DL (1988) Arthroscopic staple capsulorrhaphy for recurrent anterior shoulder instability. Arthroscopy 4:106–111

22. Morgan CD, Bodenstab AB (1987) Arthroscopic Bankart suture repair. Technique and early results. Arthroscopy 3:111–122

23. Paulos LE, Fanklin JL (1990) Arthroscopic shoulder decompression development and application. A five year experience. Am J Sports Med 8:236–244

24. Resch H (1989) Die vordere Instabilität des Schultergelenkes. Hefte Unfallheilk 202:115–163

25. Resch H, Helweg G, Zur Nedden D, Beck E (1988) Double contrast computed tomography examination techniques of habitual and recurrent shoulder dislocation. Eur J Radiol 8:6–12

26. Rockwood CA, Burkhead WZ, Brna J (1986) Subluxation of the glenohumeral joint: response to rehabilitative exercises traumatic as atraumatic instability. In: Takagishi N (ed) The shoulder. Proceedings of the Third International Conference on Surgery of the Shoulder. Professional Postgraduate Services, Fukuoka, pp 293–298

27. Seiler H (1989) Arthroskopische Stapling-Operation am Schultergelenk bei der vorderen Instabilität. Operat Orthop Traumatol 1:116–122

28. Shea K, O'Keefe R, Fulkerson JP (1990) Initial failure strength of arthroscopic Bankart suture and staple repair. Lecture AANA 9th Annual Meeting, Orlando, Florida

29. Skyhar MJ, Altcheck DW, Warren RF, Wickeewicz TL, O'Brien SJ (1988) Shoulder arthroscopy with the patient in the beach-chair position. Arthroscopy 4:265–269

30. Snyder SJ, Karzel RP, Del Pizzo W, Ferkel RD, Friedman MJ (1990) S.L.A.P. lesions of the shoulder. Arthroscopy 6:274–279

31. Wolf EM (1989) Anterior portals in shoulder arthroscopy. Arthroscopy 5:201–208

7 Arthroscopic operations in the subacromial space

7.1 Arthroscopic subacromial decompression

H. Resch, G. Sperner, and H. Thöni

Arthroscopic subacromial decompression (ASD) is a method of performing an acromioplasty as described by C.S. Neer [18] utilizing arthroscopic techniques [2, 8, 9, 11, 21]. In comparison to the open procedure, a major advantage of this method is that the deltoid muscle need not be detached. Consequently, better cosmetic results and a shorter rehabilitation time are achieved [2, 8, 12, 21].

Patients suffering from impingement syndrome with or without incomplete tears, refractory to conservative treatment, can be managed by acromioplasty alone [2, 8, 9, 18].

In patients with complete tears of the rotator cuff – with a few exceptions – open repair is recommended not only because "cuff arthropathies" [20] may develop, but also to ensure functional improvement [2].

Preoperative examination of an impingement syndrome should include a trans-scapular outlet film in addition to a.p. and axillary views. This radiograph clearly shows osteophytes on the undersurface of the AC joint and/or the anterior edge of the acromion and is suitable for the assessment of acromial morphology [3, 13, 21]. In order to obtain a precise radiograph of the undersurface of the bony roof of the shoulder, the upper part of the body must be turned to the cassette, which is placed on the lateral aspect of the shoulder, in such a way as to ensure an open anterior angle of 45–60°. Furthermore, the central beam must be directed along the spine of the scapula in posterior-anterior direction, but angled 15° caudal and aimed at the acromion (Fig. 111a and b). Acromioplasty is indicated in cases of hook-shaped acromions or where there are osteophytes on the undersurface of the acromion and AC joint, in combination with the clinical symptoms and signs of impingement syndrome (= primary impingement syndrome) [21].

If the radiographic findings of the acromion and AC joint are unremarkable, the cause of the impingement-symptoms may be situated in the joint, e.g., a hidden instability as part of a multidirectional instability or a hyperlax shoulder with or without damage to the labrum (= secondary impingement syndrome) [21] (see also Chap. 6.1). In this situation, treatment should focus on the instability rather than the impingement syndrome [2].

Ultrasonography should be performed to assess the rotator cuff [10]. If this method is not available, arthrography is indicated to establish the definite diagnosis of a rotator cuff rupture, since a complete tear will usually require reconstruction of the cuff. If the imaging techniques mentioned above do not reveal any changes in the tendon, the diagnosis of impingement syndrome should be confirmed by performing a subacromial injection test with 3 ml 2% xylocaine. A positive result, that is, the patient's pain is relieved, confirms the diagnosis. If there is no lesion in the rotator cuff, conservative treatment (therapy with stretching exercises and strengthening exercises of the internal and external rotators with the arm adducted [14]) should be commenced for a minimum duration of 6 months before performing acromioplasty.

Indications

- Impingement syndrome stage II according to Neer [19], with a history of at least one year of pain and after at least six months of conservative treatment.
- Impingement syndrome with a hook-shaped acromion or osteophyte formation on the acromion and AC joint, respectively.
- Incomplete rupture of the supraspinatus tendon on the synovial or acromial side.
- Massive rotator cuff tear in the elderly patient when performing subacromial debridement (in accordance with the open procedure according to Rockwood) [23]

Note: If there are no intact tendon structures on either the anterior or on the posterior side of the head of the humerus, acromioplasty should be avoided. In this situation the tendon remnants and bursal tissue should only be debrided, otherwise the head of the humerus may migrate antero-superiorly between the acromion and coracoid process.

Technique

Anesthesia

Arthroscopy, bursoscopy and ASD can be carried out under insufflation anesthesia as well as under regional anesthesia (interscalene block [29]). However, only general anesthesia allows hypotension. The mean arterial blood pressure should be lowered to approximately 80 mg Hg (see Chap. 2) and a systolic pressure of approximately 100 mm Hg, respectively. For this reason we usually perform ASD under general anesthesia.

Positioning and draping

Basically, there are two possible positions (see Chap. 3): (1) lateral position; (2) supine position. We have come to favor the so-called beach-chair position for virtually all arthroscopic shoulder surgery, including ASD [1, 25]).
Sterilized waterproof adhesive drapes are used to cover the area around the site of surgery. The arm, suspended in the arthroscopic elbow brace, is wrapped in a sterile "thigh stocking" (Stockinette large, Mölnlycke). Immediately after covering the area with sterile drapes, 2 ml POR 8 (ornithine-vasopressin) diluted in 18 ml saline solution are injected into

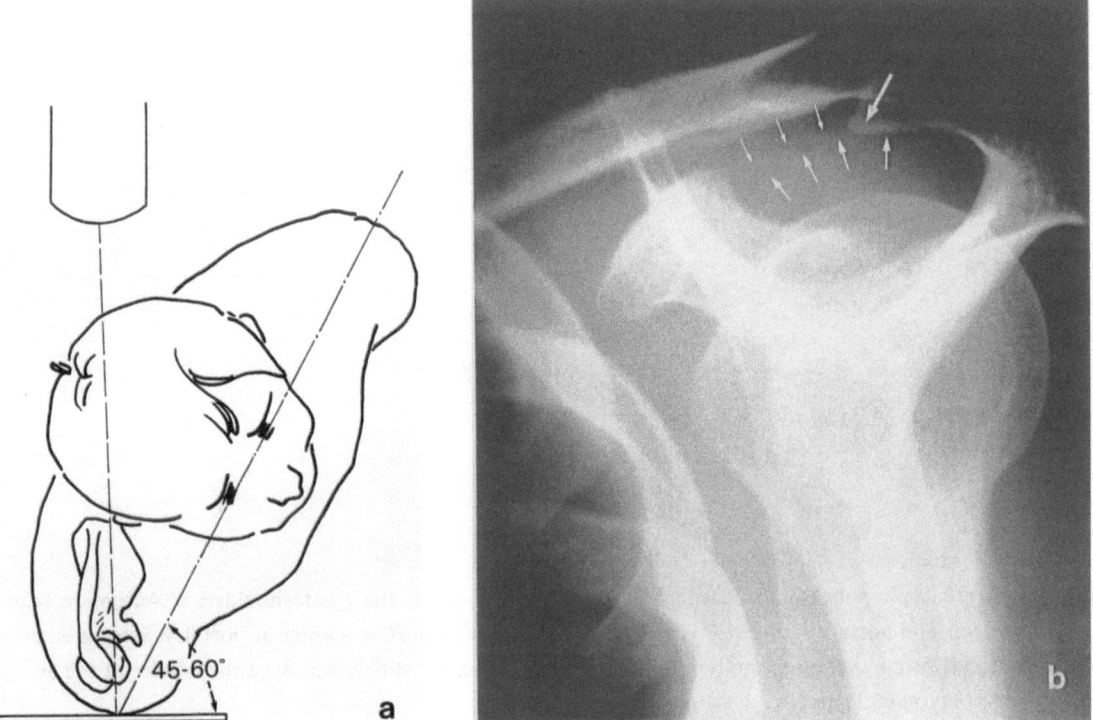

Fig. 111. Outlet view for assessment of the undersurface of the acromion and AC joint. **a** Upper part of the body inclined 45–60°; central beam is directed along the spine of the scapula with an angle of 15° caudal. **b** Hook-shaped acromion (large arrow); soft tissue shadow of rotator cuff (medium arrows) and of coracoacromial ligament (small arrows)

the subacromial space and next to the end of the acromion where the acromial branch of the thoracoacromial artery lies to provide for local vasoconstriction. Filling the bursa with fluid facilitates the introduction of a blunt trocar into the bursa. Subsequently, the acromion, the lateral end of the clavicle, the coracoid process and the coracoacromial ligament are outlined with a marking pencil on the skin in order to identify anatomic landmarks, as these may be obscured with swelling of the shoulder (edema of the soft tissue) (see Chap. 3). Furthermore, the position of the scope in the subacromial space can be determined by the markings and with the light shining through the skin.

Portals

The portals are also outlined preoperatively with a marking pencil. For ASD at least 2 or 3 portals (sometimes 4) are necessary depending on which technique is used (Fig. 112a and b).
• Posterior portal (for the arthroscope). In order to be able to use the same portal for both arthroscopy and bursoscopy, the skin incision is made 1.5 cm medial and only 1 cm inferior to the acromial angle.

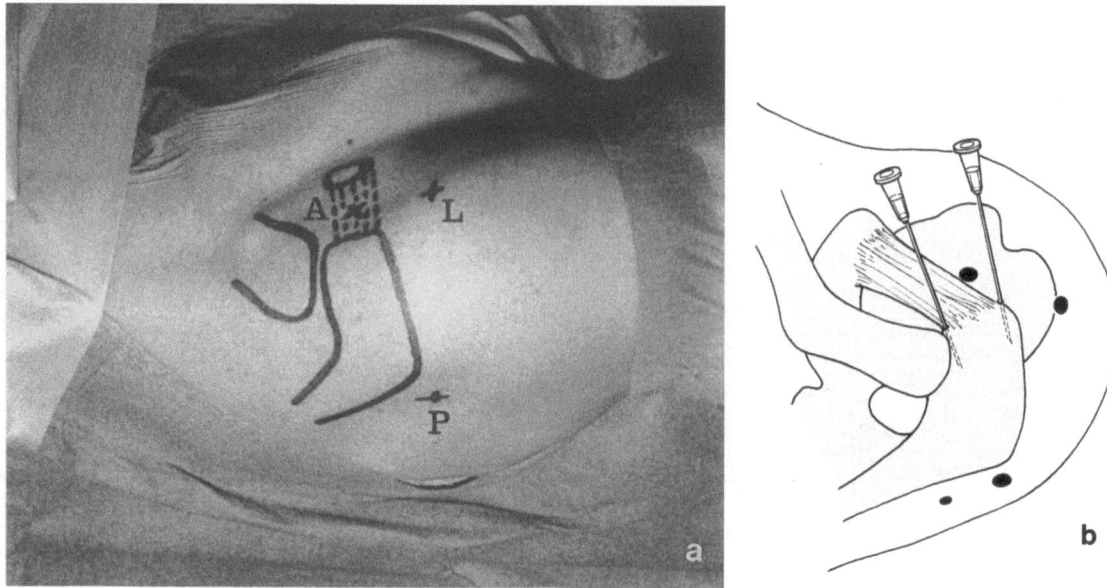

Fig. 112. Arthroscopic subacromial decompression; cranial view of the right shoulder. **a** Acromion, clavicle, coracoid process and portals outlined. *P* Posterior portal; *L* lateral portal; *A* anterior portal. **b** Schematic drawing with portals and percutaneous orientation needles for the subacromial delineation of the border of the acromion and the coracoacromial ligament

● Lateral portal (for instrumentation). This portal lies approximately 2 cm lateral to the antero-lateral corner of the acromion. All instruments except for the reciprocating file are introduced into the subacromial space via this portal.
● Anterior portal (for the reciprocating file). This is placed 1 cm anterior to the midpoint of the anterior acromial border and used for the introduction of the reciprocating file.
● Portal for the inflow cannula. If the irrigation fluid supply via the arthroscopic shaft is insufficient, an inflow cannula is inserted into the bursa 2 cm medial to the posterior portal (portal for the scope).

We use a specially manufactured "high-flow" sheath (Andre, Dornbirn, Austria) with a diameter of 6.5 mm which makes an additional inflow cannula superfluous.

Prior to every arthroscopic subacromial decompression the glenohumeral joint is inspected. On completion of this arthroscopy, the scope is removed from the sheath and a blunt trocar is introduced. The sheath is slowly withdrawn until it is felt to emerge from the joint and/or pass through the rotator cuff. When using a high-flow sheath, it is now changed. The sheath with the blunt trocar is advanced cranially under the acromion. The index finger lies on the coracoacromial ligament directly anterior to the anterior border of the acromion. The blunt trocar is advanced until it can be palpated with the finger through the ligament and the skin. The trocar is now replaced by the scope. A probe is inserted into the subacromial space through the lateral portal. If the view is obstructed by web-like tissue, this can easily be cleared with the probe. A poor view is usually caused by placement of the arthroscope in an incorrect layer of the bursa. In this situation the sheath with blunt trocar should be

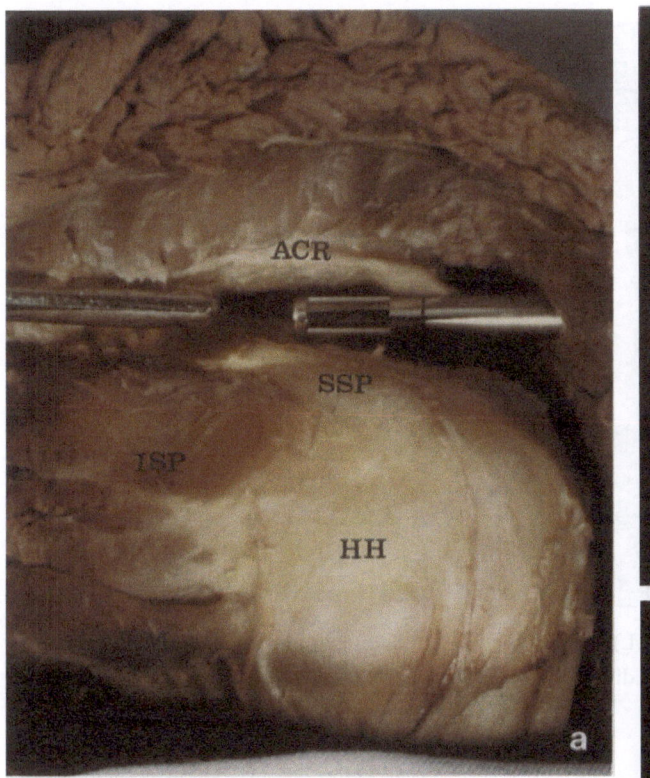

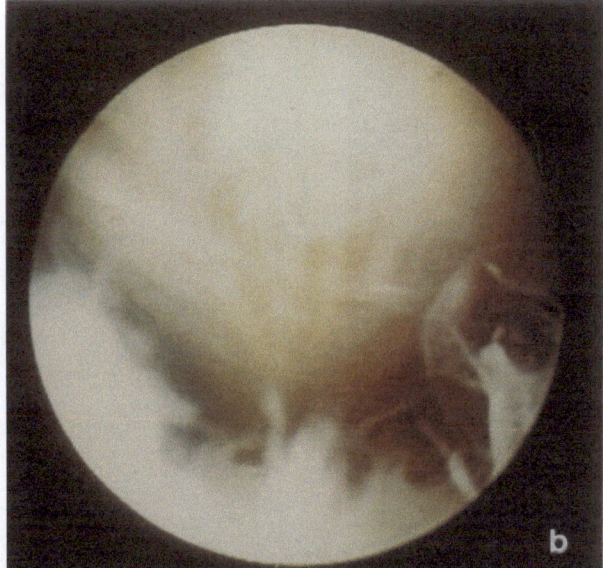

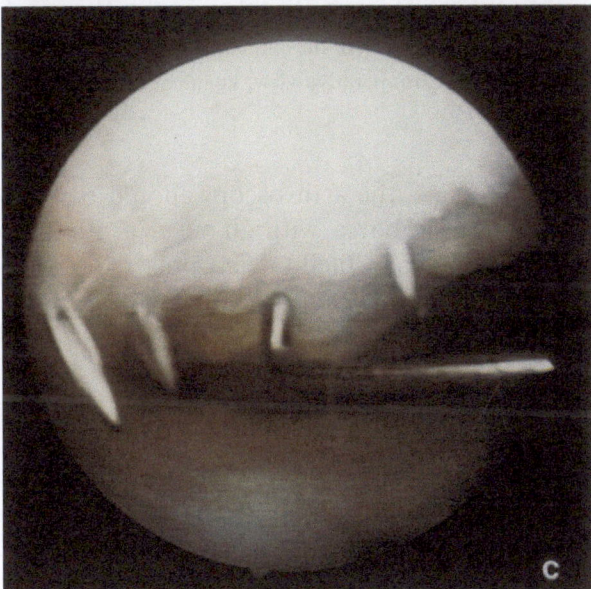

Fig. 113. Bursa shaving with synovial or full-radius resector attachment. **a** Anatomical specimen with scope and shaver in the subacromial space. *HH* Humeral head; *TM* teres minor; *ISP* infraspinatus; *SSP* supraspinatus; *ACR* acromion. **b** Coracoacromial ligament visible through bursal tissue. **c** Coracoacromial ligament delineated with two orientation needles, an additional needle (foremost needle) in the AC joint

partially withdrawn and re-inserted. Many cases require partial resection of the bursa to provide better visualization.

Bursoscopy

Insufficient vision is often caused by positioning of the arthroscope outside the bursa (as mentioned above). Before creating an artificial cavity through strong medial and lateral

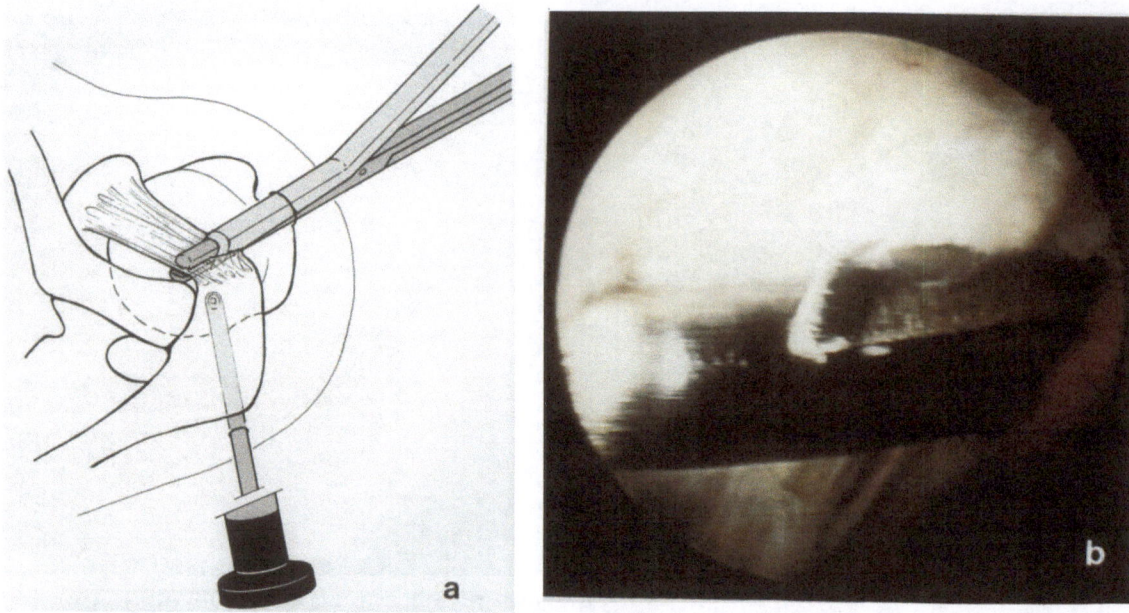

Fig. 114. Resection of the coracoacromial ligament (CAL) with sliding knife. **a** Sliding knife gliding on the ligament forceps. **b** Intraoperative view; ligament already partly divided

movements, the arthroscope should be introduced again in the hope of reaching the bursa. (Filling the bursa with 20 ml of a mixture of vasopressin and saline solution before bursoscopy greatly facilitates the insertion of the instrument.) If the view does not improve, the shaver with a 5.5 mm synovial or full-radius resector (Concept) is introduced into the subacromial space through the lateral portal and the bursa is partially resected (Fig. 113 a). The rotating blade is slowly moved in a medial and lateral direction on the rotator cuff while the assistant surgeon slowly rotates the patient's arm using the forearm which is flexed 90°. The position of the arthroscope remains largely unchanged. The shaver is then turned cranially to clear the undersurface of the coracoacromial ligament, which is already visible through the bursal tissue (Fig. 113 b). Subsequently, the upper surface of the rotator cuff is palpated with the probe. The scope and the probe remain stationary while the rotator cuff is moved by having the assistent internally and externally rotate the arm, in its 90° elbow brace.

Percutaneous marking needles at the lateral and medial borders of the acromion provide for better orientation in the subacromial space [7, 8]. These needles outline the coracoacromial ligament as well as the anterior edge of the acromion. An additional needle can be inserted through the AC joint (Fig. 113 c). The lateral border of the clavicle is identified in the subacromial space by repeated external pressure. Also, yellowish fatty tissue is often found at the undersurface of the AC joint. For the acromioplasty, the scope is rotated 180° to give a direct view of the roof of the shoulder. The light shining through the skin facilitates orientation (therefore it is important to outline the landmarks).

For the actual subacromial decompression there are basically two different approaches.

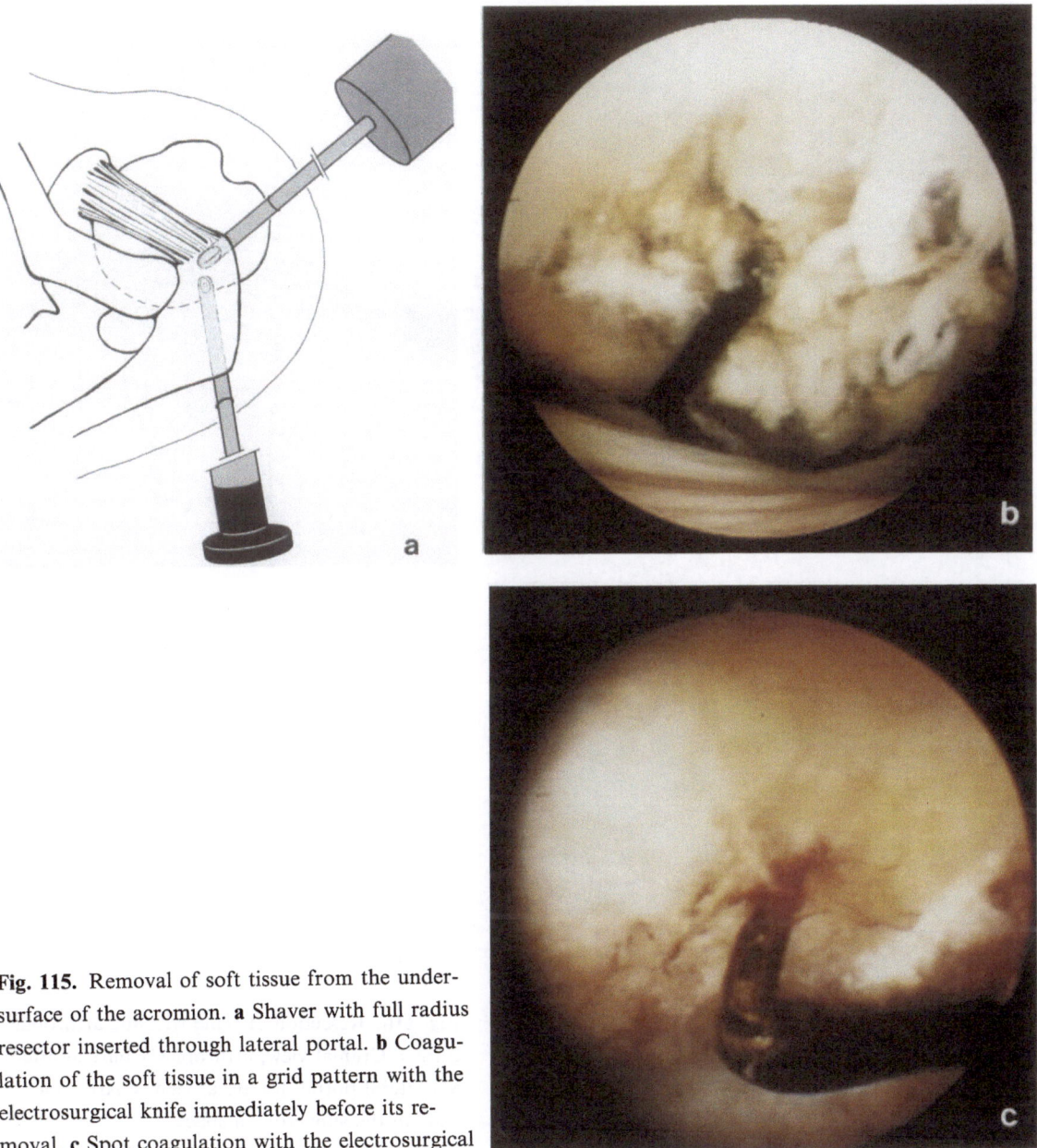

Fig. 115. Removal of soft tissue from the under-surface of the acromion. **a** Shaver with full radius resector inserted through lateral portal. **b** Coagulation of the soft tissue in a grid pattern with the electrosurgical knife immediately before its removal. **c** Spot coagulation with the electrosurgical knife

Primary division and/or resection of the coracoacromial ligament (CAL)

At ASD, first the CAL is transected and/or resected after its percutaneous delineation at the anterior edge of the acromion. Depending on the equipment available, there are two different techniques used.

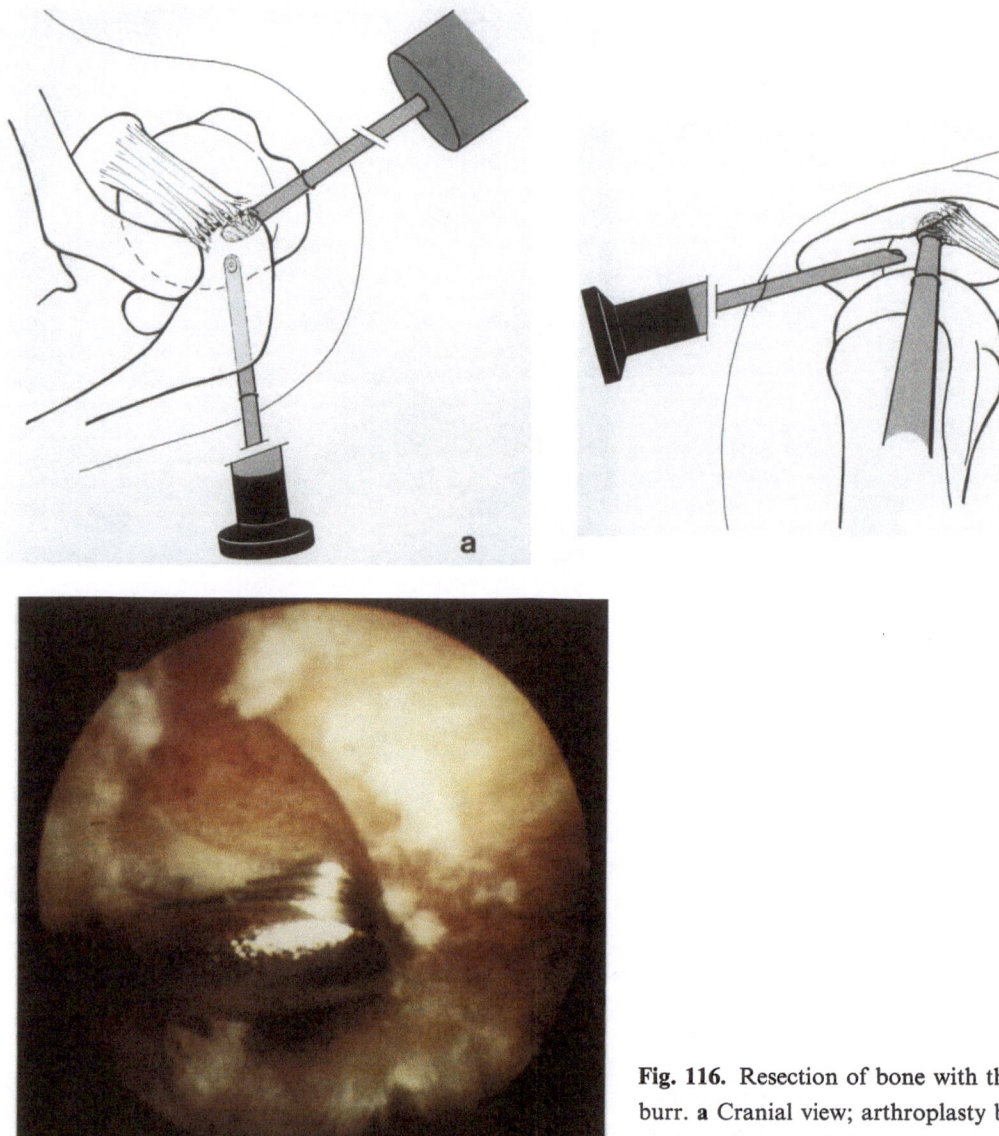

Fig. 116. Resection of bone with the arthroplasty
burr. **a** Cranial view; arthroplasty burr inserted
via lateral portal. **b** Lateral view. **c** Arthroplasty
burr in the subacromial space

Fig. 117. Resection of bone with the reciprocating file. **a** Schematic drawing in sagittal section. **b** Reciprocating file
(Micro 100, reciprocating saw; Hall/Zimmer) with file attachment. **c** Head of file. **d** Reciprocating file inserted via
anterior portal, wide suction drain in lateral universal cannula. **e** Anatomical specimen with scope and file in the
subacromial space; *TM* teres minor; *ISP* infraspinatus; *SSP* supraspinatus; *HH* humeral head; *ACR* acromion.
f Intraoperative view; filing a bony groove until desired resectional depth is reached, file is used to measure depth.
g Filed bony groove (outlined by arrows)

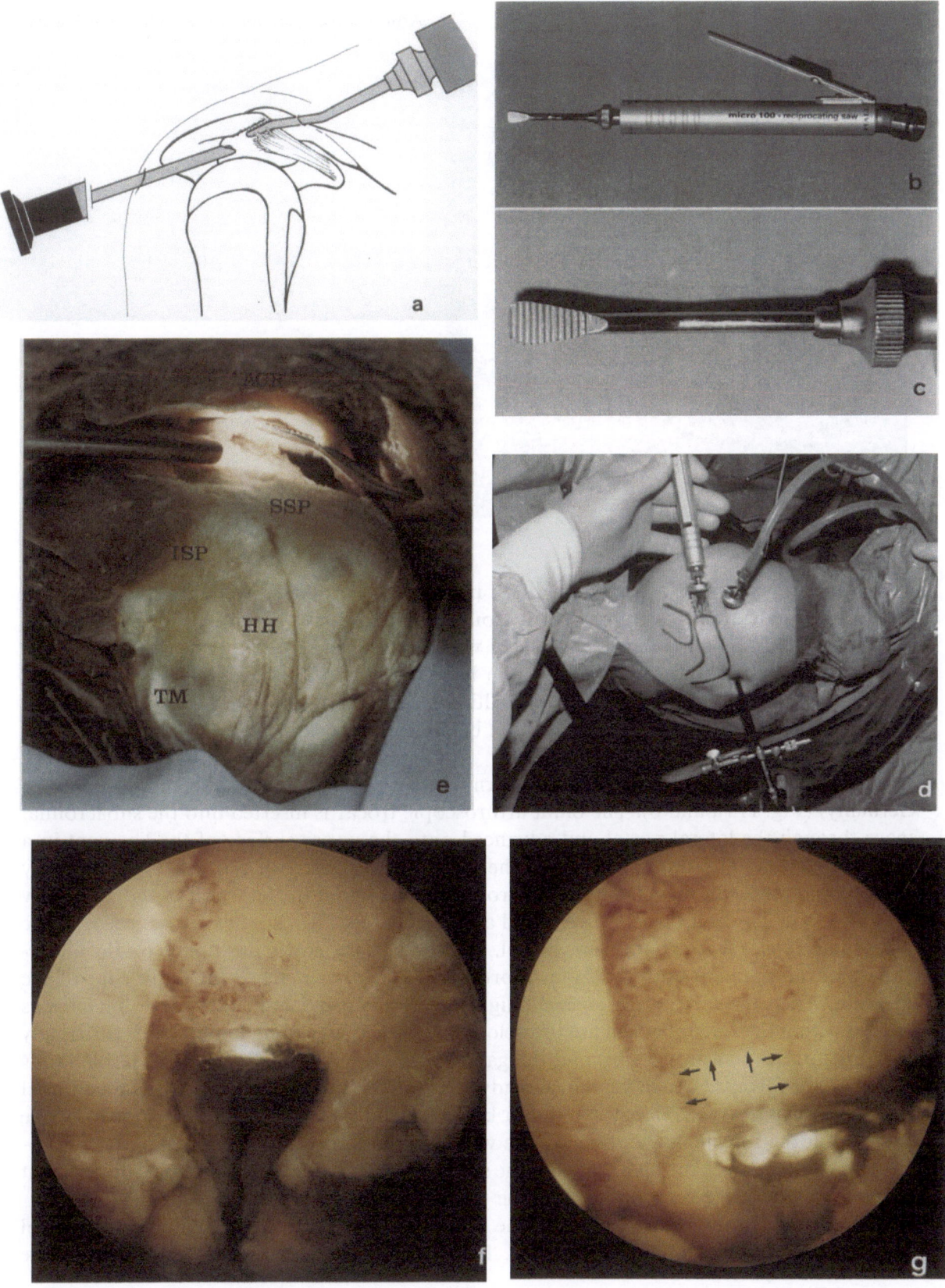

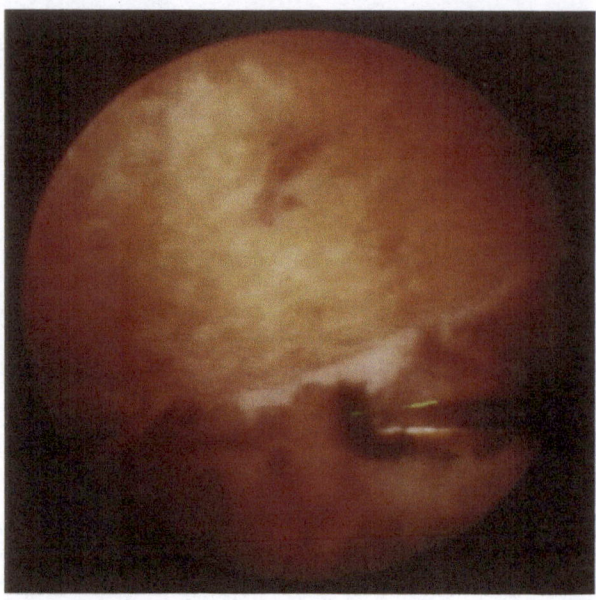

Fig. 118. Even area of resection, probe palpates thickness of the anterior border of the acromion

● Electrosurgical knife. This is introduced into the subacromial space through the lateral portal and the ligament is transected in front of the acromion from below. The anterior portion of the ligament is partially resected with the shaver (full-radius resector).

One great advantage of transecting the ligament with the electrosurgical knife is the ability to control bleeding while cutting. Although sometimes bleeding from the acromial branch of the thoracoacromial artery cannot be prevented, it can usually be stopped with the electrosurgical knife.

● Ligament forceps and U-shaped sliding knife (Leibinger, Mühlheim, Federal Republic of Germany) (Fig. 114a and b). The blunt arthroscopic trocar is inserted into the subacromial space through the lateral portal and advanced onto the upper surface of the ligament in a medial direction. The upper surface of the ligament is cleared of adjacent soft tissue by anterior and posterior movements of the trocar and prepared for insertion of the upper jaw of the forceps. The blunt trocar is removed and the ligament forceps are introduced into the subacromial space through the same portal. The forceps are slowly positioned on the under-surface of the ligament until the 3 mm shorter upper jaw has reached the outer edge of the ligament. Then the forceps are opened slightly and advanced until the whole ligament is located within the forceps which are then closed. A U-shaped sliding knife, which fits snugly over the forceps and projects beyond the gap of the forceps with its two inclined blades, is placed on the forceps outside the skin and advanced along the upper jaw into the subacromial space. The ligament is transected by both blades of the knife. The resected portion of the ligament in the forceps is then exactly the width of the forceps.

This transection of the ligament with the sliding knife has the advantage that the ligament is divided and a piece resected at the same time (approx. 0.7 cm).

One drawback in comparison with the electrosurgical knife is the inability to control bleeding during the resection procedure. If the ligament is transected too close to the acromion, the acromial branch of the thoracoacromial artery may be damaged. If necessary, bleeding has to be stopped with the electrosurgical knife afterwards.

No initial division of the coracoacromial ligament (CAL)

Initially, the CAL is visualized arthroscopically and the medial and lateral borders of the acromion are outlined with percutaneous needles. The ligament is not transected. Only after diffuse coagulation of the soft tissue on the undersurface of the acromion (see below) is the soft tissue removed. The ligament is then detached from the acromion as the edge of the acromion is carefully laid bare. The remaining part of the ligament which is still attached to the acromion is detached by the bone resection. The acromial branch of the thoracoacromial artery remains intact on the upper surface of the ligament. It is not until after resection of the bone that the ligament is partially resected with the shaver (full-radius resector).

Advantages of the technique without initial division of the ligament over the technique with initial division

Bleeding from the acromial branch of the thoracoacromial artery is less likely, since the vessel is protected on the upper side of the ligament. The bursal space remains closed for a longer period in the technique without initial transection of the ligament. This prevents the irrigation fluid from flowing into the tissues causing rapid edema. Furthermore, the irrigation fluid pressure in the subacromial space is more readily maintained to compensate for the capillary pressure (see below).

Because of its advantages, we now use the method without initial division of the CAL.

Removal of the soft tissue from the undersurface of the acromion

The shaver with a 5.5 mm full radius resector (Concept) is inserted into the subacromial space to remove the soft tissue on the undersurface of the acromion (the CAL extends 1 cm onto the undersurface of the acromion [15] and the periosteum extends dorsally). Coagulation of the soft tissue in a transverse and longitudinal direction with the electrosurgical knife facilitates and accelerates its removal with the shaver and simultaneously coagulates the periosteal vessels (Fig. 115 b–c). Consequently, there is less bleeding during the removal of the soft tissue. Complete removal of the soft tissue in the resection area is essential in order to obtain a good view during the bony resection procedure. The medial, anterior and lateral borders of the acromion must be clearly visible.

Note: When using an electrosurgical knife, sugar solutions (e.g., Resectal) are to be used instead of electrolyte solutions.

Acromioplasty

During acromioplasty the pressure in the subacromial space has to be as high as the capillary blood pressure. Usually, this is readily achieved at a mean arterial pressure of 70 to 80 mm Hg (see Chap. 2) which prevents diffuse bleeding from the cancellous bone and maintains a good view, which is crucial for precise resection of bone. The pressure in the subacromial space is either increased by a pressure controlled pump or by hanging the fluid bags extremely high via a pulley attached to the ceiling in combination with a high-flow system (see below). We use a 10 l Resectal container as a fluid bag.

The resection of bone in the antero-inferior portion of the acromion can be performed by two completely different methods.

● Motorized burr [2, 7, 9, 21] (Fig. 116a–c). An attachment with an elongated burr (arthroplasty burr 6.5 mm, Dyonics; tapered burr 6 mm or oval burr 6.5 mm, Concept) specially manufactured for acromioplasty, is inserted into the subacromial space through the lateral portal. Beginning laterally, the undersurface of the acromion is systematically burred at a relatively high rotational speed. From the beginning, the bone is resected to the desired depth. The extent of the resection has previously been determined by roentgenography (outlet view). It is usually 6–8 mm deep anteriorly and extends 1.5 to 2 cm in the posterior direction with continuously reducing depth. The thickness of the burr is used to measure the depth of the bone already resected and its length helps to gauge the extent of the resection in the posterior direction. Osteophytes of the AC joint are also removed.

Advantages of this technique: The clouded irrigation fluid is continuously drained through the motorized burr, thus ensuring a good view. This type of bone resection is also cheaper since no additional powerdriven instrument is needed. One disadvantage is that a lot of practice and precision is needed to leave the acromion smooth and without grooves.

● Reciprocating file (Fig. 117a–g). The resection of the undersurface of the acromion is not performed with a rotating burr but with a file oscillating in the longitudinal plane (Micro 100, reciprocating saw, Hall/Zimmer) (Fig. 117b). The file (part of the supplied equipment) used in place of the burr has a flat oval shape and is about 12 mm long and 6 mm wide. The length of the file can be adjusted between 6 and 8 cm. The file is inserted into the subacromial space through the anterior portal, located 1 cm anterior to the midpoint of the anterior acromial border. After the skin incision has been made, the file is advanced through the deltoid muscle in the direction of its fibers (Fig. 117a and d). At the anterior undersurface of the acromion a longitudinal groove of the width of the reciprocating file is made to the desired resectional depth under vision. The extent of the resection has already been determined by roentgenography (outlet view). The thickness of the file (approx. 2 mm) is used to measure the resectional depth (normally 2 to 3 times the thickness of the file at the anterior edge of the acromion) and its length is used to measure the posterior extent of the resection (Fig. 117e–g). Subsequently, the rest of the undersurface of the acromion, starting with the lateral portion and moving in a medial direction as far as the AC joint, is systematically resected to the desired level. Osteophytes on the AC joint are also removed. A wide suction cannula is placed in the universal cannula in the lateral portal. A universal cannula with suction equipment (Acufex) to which a tube can be directly connected is an advantage. If a pressure controlled pump is not used, the assistant surgeon controls the visibility in the subacromial space by opening and closing the suction tube. Before completion of the acromioplasty, the probe is used to detect irregularities on the undersurface of the acromion and in particular along its edges; these are then removed under vision. The thickness of the anterior acromial edge is assessed with the probe (Fig. 118). On completion of the acromioplasty, a suction drain is placed in the subacromial space through the arthroscopic sheath and the incisions are closed.

Advantages of the technique: Creation of a smooth and even resection area; accurate control of the extent of bone resection; the reciprocating file rarely damages the soft tissue, even if the file comes in direct contact with it. Drawbacks: If the reciprocating file hits the end of the scope, the latter may be damaged. An additional powerdriven instrument (reciprocating file) is needed. Because the clouded irrigation fluid is not continuously drained vision is sometimes not as good as in the case where the burr is used.

Control of bleeding in the subacromial space (SAS)

The most important measure to control bleeding in the SAS is by compensating for the capillary blood pressure with the irrigation fluid pressure. This can be achieved by the following measures.

● Controlled hypotension: the mean arterial blood pressure of the patient should be lowered to 70–80 mm Hg (about 100 mm Hg systolic pressure). This is, however, only possible in the healthy patient under general anesthesia. The reduction of systemic blood pressure is the most important measure to control bleeding in the SAS.

● Increasing pressure in the subacromial space: this is achieved by using a pressure controlled pump or hanging the fluid bag extremely high by means of a pulley attached to the ceiling. The subacromial space is irrigated via a high-flow system (extra-wide tube couplings, high-flow sheath, or additional inflow cannula). We now routinely use a 10 l Resectal container as fluid bag.

Further measures include:

● Meticulous cautery of vessels with the electrosurgical knife, as well as coagulation of the soft tissue on the undersurface of the acromion before removal. If no electrosurgical knife is available, the irrigation fluid must be kept clear by repeated rinsing and draining which is very time consuming (without an electrosurgical knife ASD is almost impossible).

● Injection of ornithine-vasopressin (2 ml POR 8 diluted in 18 ml NaCl) into the subacromial space and, particularly, to the end of the acromion (acromial branch of the thoracoacromial artery) before bursoscopy to provide for local vasoconstriction. This can only be regarded as an additional measure. (The local use of this amount of POR 8 produces minimal or no increase in the systemic blood pressure.) Filling the bursa with fluid also facilitates the correct insertion of the sheath.

Postoperative management following ASD

Immediately after surgery the arm is placed in a sling. On the first postoperative day the drain is removed. By this time, usually the soft tissue edema has completely disappeared. Simultaneously, passive motion in all planes is begun. Four days after surgery active assisted motion is commenced. The patient now also begins strengthening exercises (isometric exercises) of the external and internal rotators with the upper arm in an adducted position [14]. Thus, the muscles acting as depressors of the head of the humerus are strengthened. Overhead sports activities should be avoided for at least 3 months.

Patient information

Arthroscopic subacromial decompression is a surgical technique which causes a minimal amount of trauma. Nevertheless, its success relies heavily on the ability to control bleeding as this is crucial for good visualization of the subacromial space. In case of heavy bleeding it may become necessary to change to an open procedure and the patient should be informed of this preoperatively. When the surgeon is inexperienced, the success rate of the arthroscopic method is somewhat lower than that of an open procedure; consequently, if the arthroscopic decompression is unsuccessful an open procedure may later become necessary. During ASD neurological damage is very unlikely.

Results after arthroscopic subacromial decompression

From 1987 to 1991 168 patients with stage II and III impingement syndrome underwent arthroscopic subacromial decompression. In 64 patients bone resection was performed with the reciprocating file and in 104 patients the arthroplasty burr was used. The first 50 patients (32 patients, reciprocating file and 18 patients, arthroplasty burr) had a follow-up examination according to the UCLA Shoulder Rating Scale [8]. In accordance with this scale, pain and function are rated from 1–10, active range of motion, strength and patient satisfaction are rated on a scale of 1–5. The maximum total score is 35 points. At a mean follow-up of 19 months (12–34 months), twenty-six percent of the patients had excellent results (32–35 points), 60% good (28–32 points), 8% fair (21–28 points) and 6% poor results (<21 points). In accordance with the rating system described by Neer and Ellman [8, 18], 86% of the patients had satisfactory results (≥28 points) and 14% had unsatisfactory results (<28 points). Twenty-eight percent of the patients were satisfied and 12% were not satisfied with their results. Of the patients with incomplete tears and small complete tears (<1 cm) 83% had satisfactory results, which were results similar to those of the patients without tears (88% with satisfactory results). When comparing patients with impingement syndrome stage II and III, the results were also quite similar (86% satisfactory results at stage II and 83% satisfactory results at stage III). The cited results are comparable to those of other authors, especially those authors who used the same rating system (Ellman 88% satisfactory results [8], Esch 85% satisfactory results [9]). Altcheck [2] and Paulos [21] also report similar results. The results after ASD are similar with those after open acromioplasty [13, 18, 26]. After one week 34% of our patients had returned to work and 63% after one month. Paulos [21] reported that 59% of his patients had returned to work after one week, while Altcheck [2] reported that 89% of his patients had returned to work in the first week after discharge from hospital. One possible explanation for the apparent late return to work of our patients is the high proportion (47%) involved in physical labor. While Tibone [27] reported that only 43% of his patients returned to their former sports activities after open acromioplasty, 70% of our patients did so after ASD, while Altcheck [2] and Paulos [21] reported figures of 76% and 83%, respectively. The rapid functional recovery is attributed to the minimal postoperative morbidity and to the fact that the deltoid muscle is not detached.

7.2 Arthroscopic subacromial calcium removal

H. Resch, G. Sperner, and K. Golser

Calcific deposits in the tendons of the rotator cuff are very frequent. However, they are usually asymptomatic and are often only discovered as coincidental findings. Their composition varies, consisting of calcium phosphate, calcium oxalate, calcium carbonate and hydroxyapatite [4, 22]. Somewhat surprisingly though, even very small, normally asymptomatic calcifications may cause very severe and lasting pains in the course of a shoulder injury without there being any macroscopically visible change. One reason for this may be a traumatically induced local inflammation. Often the calcific deposits are unjustly thought to be the cause of pain when there is no other visible reason for the symptoms mentioned. Calcific deposits in the rotator cuff can be responsible for shoulder complaints in two ways:

(1) Long-term asymptomatic calcific deposits may suddenly liquefy, break through the tendon surface and flow into the subacromial bursa. The consistency of the calcium during this process is milky and creamlike. During the discharge a sudden severe inflammatory reaction is seen, which lasts from 3 to 5 days and then quickly subsides again [6, 24]. The acute inflammatory phase, which can be very painful and which may coincide with an externally visible inflammatory swelling, justifies a subacromial injection of cortisone to relieve the inflammation. Ice packs also alleviate the pain. It is not possible to say in advance how long the subsequent pain-free interval will last (see also Chap. 5).

(2) Calcific deposits can increase in size to such an extent that not only do they reach the surface of the tendon but make it bulge outwards (Fig. 119a). Due to their size, these calcific deposits lead to impaction symptoms under the acromion when they are located in the region of the supraspinatus tendon, thus resulting in an impingement syndrome [24]. If conservative treatment is unsuccessful, operative removal is required.

Radiography is usually sufficient for establishing the diagnosis of a calcific tendinitis. For better localization we recommend a.p. views with the arm in 60° of external rotation (supraspinatus tendon) and 60° of internal rotation (infraspinatus tendon). Ultrasonography is very helpful for localizing the deposits, provided that the surgeon is experienced in this field. Very compact calcium accumulations, however, cause sonographic shadows behind the calcifications [10] (Fig. 119b). Only calcific deposits which touch the surface of the tendon or make it bulge out can be removed arthroscopically, as they are otherwise very difficult to locate. On an a.p. X-ray of good quality the soft tissue shadow of the tendon can often be seen and assessed. Conservative treatment (physiotherapy) should always precede the surgical intervention. Preoperatively, X-rays should be taken, as calcific deposits can change their position and shape within weeks.

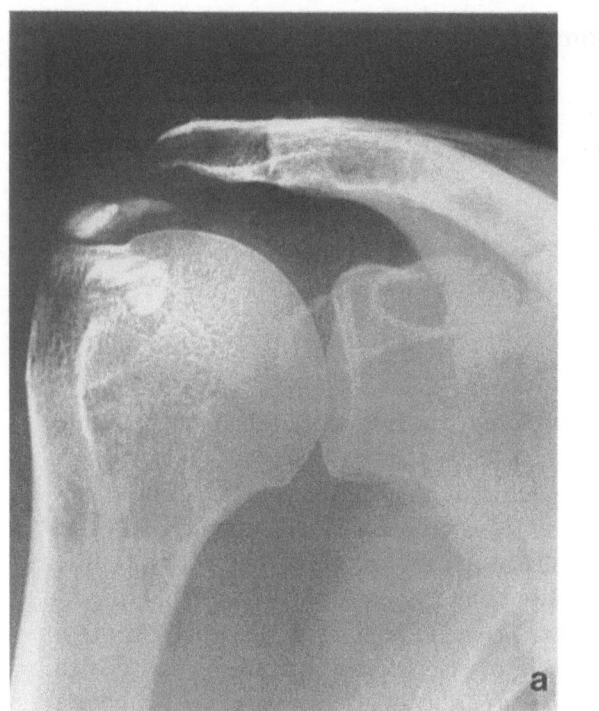
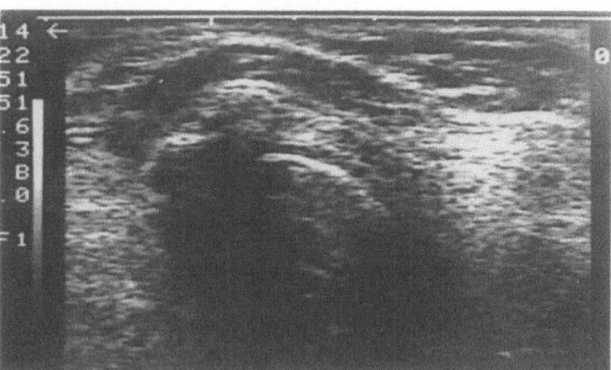
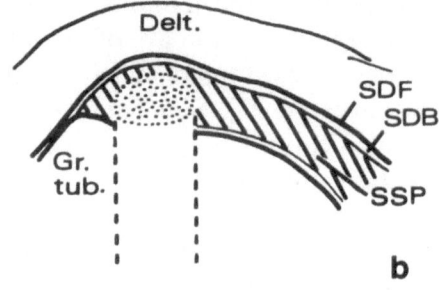

Fig. 119. Calcific deposit. **a** A.P.-view with the arm in 60° of external rotation shows compact calcific deposit in full size. **b** Sonogram (above) of the same deposit with schematic drawing (below); surface of tendon protrudes in a humplike manner; sonographic shadow behind the deposit. *SDF* Subdeltoid fascia; *SDB* subdeltoid bursa; *SSP* supraspinatus tendon; *Gr. tub.* greater tuberosity; *Delt.* deltoid muscle

Technique

Anesthesia, positioning and portals are the same as in the bursoscopy already described (Chaps. 5 and 7.1). An anterior portal is only required if an additional acromioplasty with a reciprocating file is planned.

Bursoscopy

This procedure does not differ from the technique described above (Chaps. 5 and 7.1). If the calcific deposits protrude in a humplike manner, they are easily localized and extensive bursa shaving is normally not required. Generally, it is necessary to resect the layer of the subdeltoid bursa covering the rotator cuff with a shaver (5.5 mm full-radius resector attachment, Concept). This facilitates detection of the deposit which shines through the tendon surface. By carefully scraping the surface with a probe, the calcium usually appears as a viscous mass, sometimes as crumbly lumps (Fig. 120a and b). Careful curettage with the probe normally suffices as therapy, sometimes a small sharp spoon must be introduced through the lateral

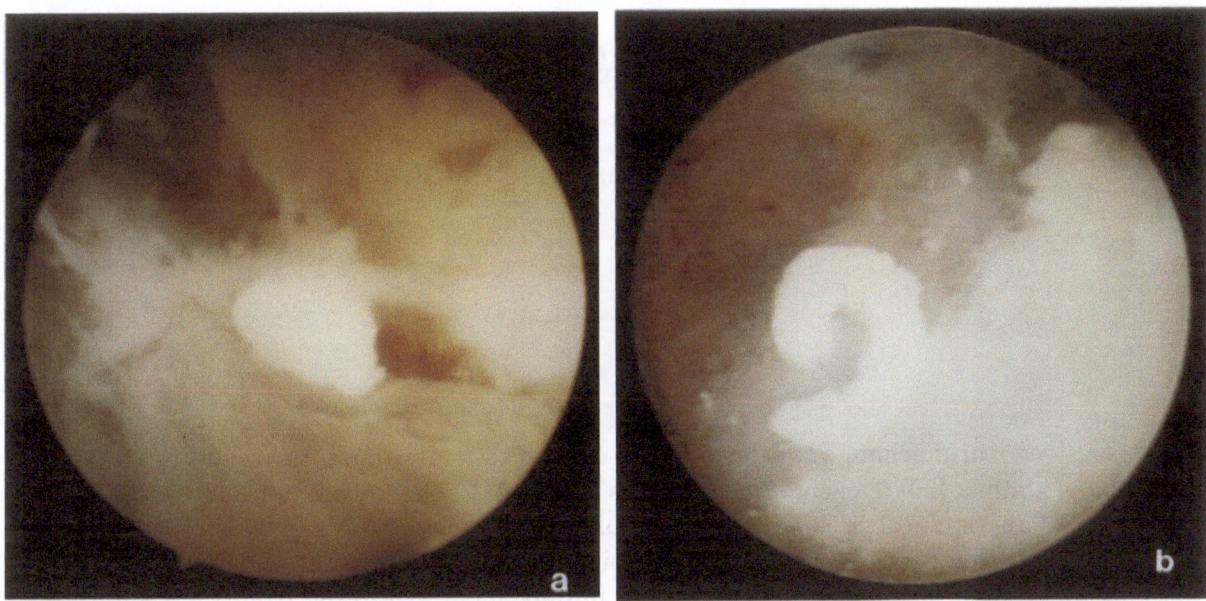

Fig. 120. Intraoperative pictures of calcium removal after scraping open the tendon surface. **a** Calcium flows out as a crumbly mass. **b** Calcium flows out as a doughy mass

portal (in case of a crumbly consistency). Only as much calcium should be removed as can be done without destroying the tendon. Any residual calcium between the tendon fibres is often reabsorbed with the hyperemia following the operation. In case of restriction of movement in the shoulder joint, arthroscopic subacromial decompression (acromioplasty) is usually carried out in addition to removal. Experience has shown that pain relief and restoration of function is achieved more rapidly this way.

7.3 Arthroscopic resection of the lateral end of the clavicle

H. Resch, H. Thöni, and R. Butorac

Degenerative arthritic changes of the acromio-clavicular joint are frequent, and usually the sequelae of trauma [30]. Degenerative arthritis of the AC-joint must be differentiated from osteolysis of the lateral end of the clavicle. Osteolytic changes are not usually caused by trauma but by repetitive overuse of the AC-joint (e.g., weight-lifting) [5]. In a few cases, it may be difficult to distinguish a subacromial impingement syndrome from the symptoms caused by degenerative arthritis or osteolysis of the clavicular end. In case of doubt, the local anesthetic test is helpful in distinguishing the symptoms. This test should first be carried out in the subacromial space (impingement sign according to Neer [19]) and then in the AC-joint. This order should be followed since the joint cavity is sometimes difficult to locate in the degenerative arthritic AC-joint, and the local anesthetic may leak into the area around the AC-joint and the subacromial space. If the inferior joint capsule is perforated, the local anesthetic may accidentally be injected into the subacromial space, resulting in a false test result. For arthroscopic resection of the lateral end of the clavicle it is important to determine whether the AC-joint is stable or unstable. This is assessed by displacement of the lateral end of the clavicle in the vertical plane by comparative radiological AP-views of both shoulders, with traction being applied to both arms. If there is instability, resection of the lateral end of the clavicle alone should not be performed. In this case an additional syndesmoplasty is required to stabilize the lateral end of the clavicle. For this purpose we commonly use the coracoacromial ligament (operation according to Weaver and Dunn [28]).

If there is an impingement syndrome in combination with a degenerative arthritis of the AC-joint, we recommend the combined arthroscopic subacromial decompression and resection of the lateral end of the .clavicle, with the acromioplasty being performed first (see below). For arthroscopic resection of the AC-joint, it is necessary to distinguish between osteolysis and degenerative arthritis.

(1) Degenerative arthritis (Fig. 121) has a hard sclerosed subchondral zone. Removal of the lateral end of the clavicle with the rotating burr (arthroplasty burr; Concept) or reciprocating file (reciprocating file; Hall/Zimmer) is very time-consuming, therefore an open resection through a small incision directly over the AC-joint should be considered.

(2) Osteolysis (Fig. 122a and b) is characterized by a cystic-porotic change of the acromial end of the clavicle. Removal can be accomplished easily and rapidly with the rotating burr (arthroplasty burr) as well as with the reciprocating file.

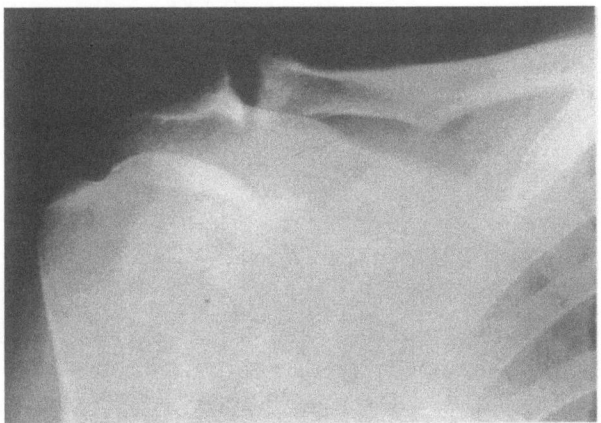

Fig. 121. Degenerative arthritic change of the AC-joint

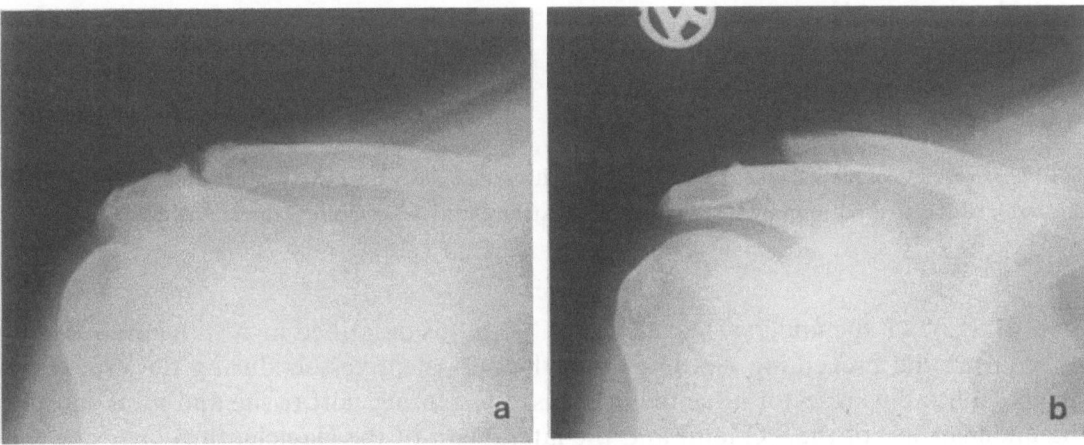

Fig. 122. Osteolytic change of the lateral end of the clavicle. **a** Before arthroscopic resection. **b** After arthroscopic resection

Technique

If resection of the lateral end of the clavicle is scheduled in combination with an arthroscopic subacromial decompression (ASD), the acromioplasty is to be performed first (see Chap. 7.1), as the caudal joint capsule and the soft tissue from the undersurface of the acromion can be removed at the same time. The bevelled acromion also facilitates access to the AC-joint.

Anesthesia, positioning and portals are the same as for bursoscopy (Chaps. 5 and 7.1). The yellow fatty tissue which is almost always present on the undersurface of the AC-joint, facilitates localization of the AC-joint. The AC-joint is readily identified by exerting external pressure on the lateral end of the clavicle and observation of moves. The electrosurgical knife, which is inserted into the subacromial space through the lateral portal, is used to cauterize

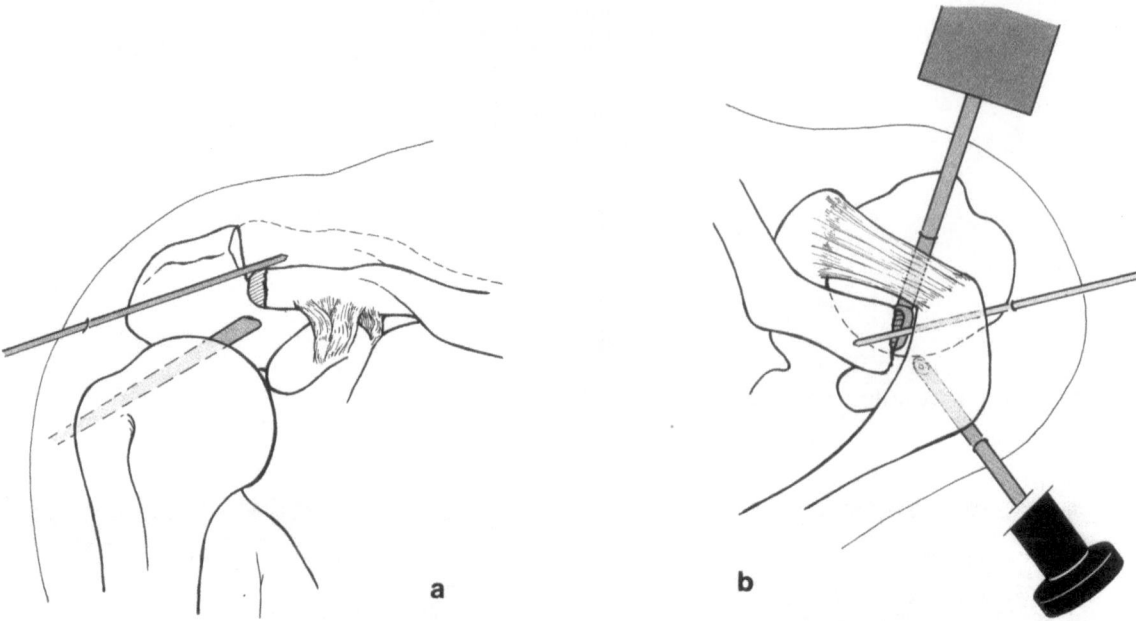

Fig. 123. Resection of the lateral end of the clavicle with arthroplasty burr (6.5 mm). **a** End of clavicle maintained in inferior dislocation position by Kirschner wire. **b** Arthroplasty burr inserted directly anterior to AC-joint

the soft tissue on the undersurface of the AC-joint (as described in ASD), hereby facilitating its removal and preventing bleeding from the periosteal vessels during the procedure. The shaver (full radius resector attachment) is used to remove soft tissue and joint capsule from the undersurface of the AC-joint and the lateral end of the clavicle, thus exposing the joint cavity. If possible, the anterior and posterior parts of the capsule should also be removed in order to mobilize the lateral end of the clavicle.

The resection itself, which should measure about 1 cm [17], can, like ASD, be performed in two ways.

Arthroplasty burr

Careful removal of the inferior capsule of the AC-joint, including its anterior and posterior margins, mobilizes the lateral end of the clavicle to such an extent that it can be pressed down for almost its entire width with the thumb. From about 2 cm behind the lateral portal a 2 mm Kirschner wire is advanced percutaneously under the acromion until it reaches the upper surface of the lateral end of the clavicle, which maintains the clavicle in an inferiorly displaced position (Fig. 123a). If the joint is very taut and acromioplasty has not been performed, it is usually necessary to resect a few millimeters of bone from the medial undersurface of the acromion in order to be able to slip the pin over the lateral end of the clavicle. Residual portions of the articular disc which become visible are now removed with the forceps. If there is osteolytic change, resection of the lateral end of the clavicle can be

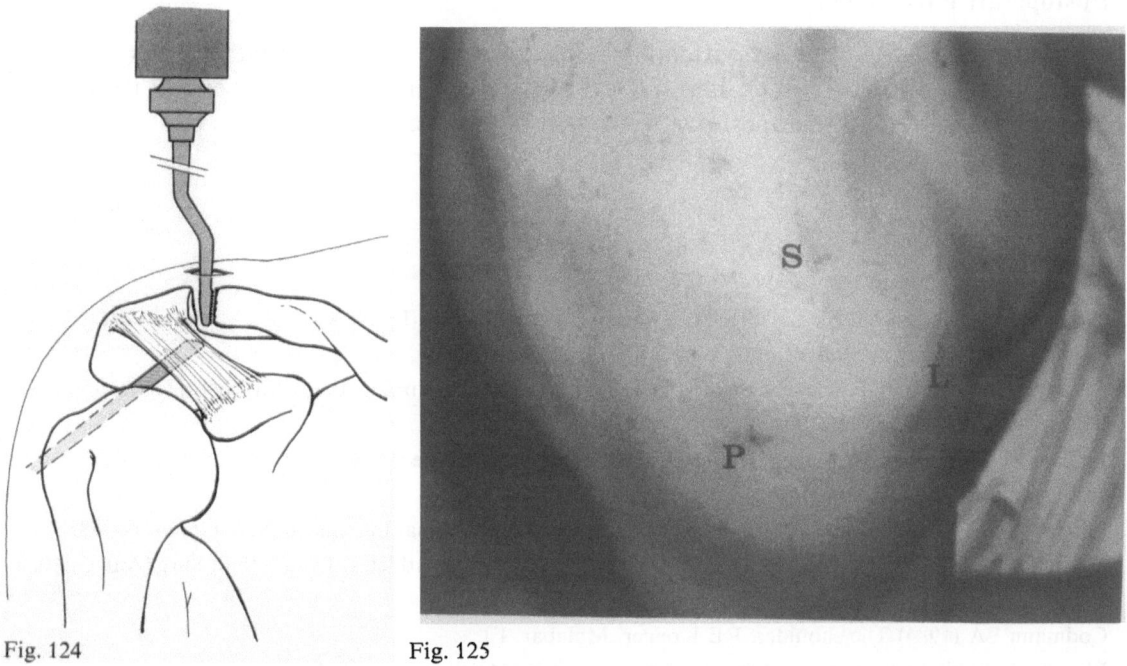

Fig. 124   Fig. 125

Fig. 124. Resection of lateral end of clavicle with reciprocating file through cranial portal; scope from posterior

Fig. 125. Right shoulder after resection of the lateral end of the clavicle from a cranial direction with reciprocating file. *P* Posterior portal (scope), *L* lateral portal (shaver), *S* superior portal (file)

performed through the lateral portal, as the rotating burr does not need to be pressed against the soft bone. A sclerotic clavicle usually requires a new portal directly anterior to the AC-joint. When inserting it through this portal, the burr is brought parallel to the joint surface of the lateral end of the clavicle, which creates a better working surface for the burr (Fig. 123 b). The length (approx. 10 mm) and the thickness (approx. 6.5 mm) of the burr are used to measure the extent of the resection (approx. 1 cm).

Reciprocating file

A skin incision measuring approx. 1 cm is made cranial to, and directly above the AC-joint and at right angle to it. When using this portal, residual soft tissue (residual disc) is removed with the forceps (rangeur). Subsequently, the reciprocating file is introduced into the joint cavity from a cranial direction and 1 cm of the lateral end of the clavicle is filed off (Fig. 124). The filing procedure is observed from the subacromial space through the scope. The width of the file serves as a guideline for the extent of the resection (Fig. 125).

Note: Before completing the resection, the traction weight must be removed from the arm, as it further widens the resection gap!

Postoperative treatment

When performing ASD together with an AC-resection, the postoperative treatment is determined by the acromioplasty (see Chap. 7.1). If only resection of the lateral end of the clavicle is performed, no special postoperative treatment is required.

References

1. Altcheck DW, Warren RF, Skyhar MK (1990) Shoulder arthroscopy. In: Rickwood CA, Matsen FA (eds) The shoulder. WB Saunders, Philadelphia, pp 258–277
2. Altcheck DW, Warren RF, Wickiewicz TL, Skyhar MJ, Ortiz G, Schwartz E (1990) Arthroscopic acromioplasty. J Bone Joint Surg [Am] 72:1198–1207
3. Bigliani LU, Morrison DS, Aprol EW (1986) The morphology of the acromion and its relationship to rotator cuff tears. Orthop Trans 10:216
4. Bosworth B (1941) Calcium deposits in the shoulder and subacromial bursitis. JAMA 116:2477–2482
5. Cahill ER (1982) Osteolysis of the distal part of the clavicle in male athletes. J Bone Joint Surg [Am] 64:1053–1058
6. Codmann EA (1984) The shoulder. RE Kreiger, Malabar, FL
7. Ellman H (1985) Arthroscopic subacromial decompression. Orthop Trans 9:48
8. Ellmann H (1987) Arthroscopic subacromial decompression: analysis of one- to three-year results. Arthroscopy 3:173–181
9. Esch JC, Ozerkis LR, Helgager JA, et al (1988) Arthroscopic subacromial decompression: results according to the degree of rotator cuff tear. Arthroscopy 4:241–249
10. Furtschegger A, Resch H (1988) Value of ultrasonography in preoperative diagnosis of rotator cuff tears and postoperative follow-up. Eur J Radiol 8:69–75
11. Gartsman GM, Blair ME, Noble PC, Bennett JB, Tullos HS (1988) Arthroscopic subacromial decompression. An anatomical study. Am J Sports Med 16:48–50
12. Johnson LL (1987) The shoulder joint. An arthroscopist's perspective of anatomy and pathology. Clin Orthop 223:113–125
13. McShane RB, Lainberry CF, Fenlin JM (1987) Conservative anterior acromioplasty. Clin Orthop 223:137–144
14. Matsen AF, Arntz CT (1990) Subacromial impingement. In: Rockwood CA, Matsen FA (eds) The shoulder. WB Saunders, Philadelphia, pp 623–646
15. Matthews LS, Fadale PD (1989) Subacromial anatomy for the arthroscopist. Arthroscopy 5:36–40
16. Morrison DS, Bigliani LU (1987) Roentgenographic analysis of acromial morphology and its relationship to rotator cuff tears. Orthop Trans 11:439
17. Mumford EB (1941) Acromioclavicular dislocation. A new operative treatment. J Bone Joint Surg 23:799–802
18. Neer CS II (1972) Anterior acromioplasty for the chronic impingement syndrome in the shoulder: a preliminary report. J Bone Joint Surg [Am] 54:41–50
19. Neer CS II (1983) Impingement lesions. Clin Orthop 173:70–77
20. Neer CS, Craig EV, Fukuda H (1983) Cuff-tear arthropathy. J Bone Joint Surg [Am] 62:1232–1244
21. Paulos LE, Franklin JL (1990) Arthroscopic shoulder decompression development and application. A five year experience. Am J Sports Med 18:235–244
22. Resnick CS, Resnick D (1983) Crystal deposition disease. Semin Arthritis Rheum 2:39 B

23. Rockwood CA Jr (1986) The management of patients with massive defects in the rotator cuff. Presented at Mid-America Orthopaedic Association Meeting, Orlando, Florida, April 2–6, 1986

24. Rowe CR (1988) The shoulder. Churchill Livingstone, New York

25. Skyhar MJ, Altcheck DW, Warren RF, Wickiewicz TL, O'Brien SJ (1988) Shoulder arthroscopy with the patient in the beach-chair position. Arthroscopy 4:265–269

26. Thorling J, Bjerneld H, Hallin G, Hovelins L, Hagg O (1985) Acromioplasty for impingement syndrome. Acta Orthop Scand 56:147–148

27. Tibone JE, Jobe FW, Kerlan RK, Carter VS, Shields CL, Lombardi SJ, Yocum LA (1985) Shoulder impingement syndrome in athletes treated by an anterior acromioplasty. Clin Orthop 198:134–140

28. Weaver KL, Dunn HK (1972) Treatment of acromioclavicular injuries, especially complete acromio-clavicular separations. J Bone Joint Surg [Am] 54:1187–1197

29. Winnie AP (1970) Interscalene branchial plexus block. Anesth Analg 49:455–466

30. Wirth CJ, Breitner S (1984) Die Resektion des acromialen Claviculaendes bei der Schultereckgelenkarthrose. Z Orthop 122:208–212

Subject index

Luigi Celli (ed.)

The Shoulder

Periarticular Degenerative Pathology

(Current Concepts in Orthopaedic Surgery)

Translated by Sylvia Notini

1990. With 124 Figures (190 single illustrations). 138 pages.
Cloth DM168,-, öS 1176,-. ISBN 3-211-82219-4

Prices are subject to change without notice

In the first part of this volume two basic points are presented: an in-depth study of the biomechanics and physiopathology of the joint complex of the shoulder and improved diagnostic methods which have allowed for a clearer identification of various pathologies. In the second part of this volume it is shown how the improvement in physiopathological knowledge and diagnostic methods has resulted in finer surgical methods. This volume will be of interest to all physicians in the field of orthopaedic surgery, radiology, rheumatology and rehabilitation.

Jointly published by Springer-Verlag Wien New York and Aulo Gaggi Editore, Bologna
Sole distribution rights: Springer-Verlag Wien New York

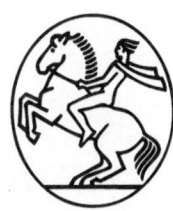

Springer-Verlag Wien New York